CBS—Quick Medical Examination Review Series

RADIOLOGY

FIFTEENTH EDITION

Edited by :

DR. M.S. BHATIA (MD, Dip. WPA, MNAMS)
Professor & Head, Department of Psychiatry
University College of Medical Sciences
&
Guru Teg Bahadur Hospital,
Dilshad Garden, Delhi - 110095.

Previously at :
Maulana Azad Medical College and Associated Hospitals, New Delhi.
&
Lady Hardinge Medical College and Associated Hospitals, New Delhi

Contributing Editor :
DR. NIRMALJIT KAUR (MD)
Senior Specialist, Department of Microbiology
Dr. R.M.L. Hospital
New Delhi - 110001

Previously at :
LHMC & Smt. S.K. Hospital, New Delhi

CBS

CBS PUBLISHERS & DISTRIBUTORS PVT. LTD.

NEW DELHI • BANGALORE • PUNE • COCHIN • CHENNAI (INDIA)

DEDICATED TO
READERS WHO READ, UNDERSTAND
&
RECIPROCATE

ISBN : 978-81-239-1834-1

First Edition : 1992
Second Edition : 1993
Third Edition : 1994
Fourth Edition : 1995
Fifth Edition : 1996
Sixth Edition : 1997
Seventh Edition : 1998
Eighth Edition : 1999
Ninth Edition : 2000
Tenth Edition : 2001
Eleventh Edition : 2002
Twelveth Edition : 2003
Thirteenth Edition : 2004
Fourteenth Edition : 2005
Fifteenth Edition : 2010

Published by Satish Kumar Jain and produced by V.K. Jain for
CBS Publishers & Distributors Pvt. Ltd.,
CBS Plaza, 4819/XI Prahlad Street, 24 Ansari Road, Daryaganj,
New Delhi - 110002, India.
e-mail: cbspubs@vsnl.com, cbspubs@airtelmail.in, delhi@cbspd.com
Website: www.cbspd.com

Branches:

- ***Bangalore:*** Seema House, 2975, 17th Cross, K.R. Road, Bansankari 2nd Stage, Bangalore - 560070
  Fax: 080-26771680 • e-mail: bangalore@cbspd.com
- ***Pune:*** Shaan Brahmha Complex, 631/632, Basement, Appa Balwant Chowk, Budhwar Peth, Next to Ratan Talkies, Pune - 411002
  Fax: 020-24464059 • e-mail: pune@cbspd.com
- ***Cochin:*** 36/14, Kalluvilakam, Lissie Hospital Road, Cochin - 682018, Kerala • e-mail: cochin@cbspd.com
- ***Chennai:*** 20, West Park Road, Shenoy Nagar, Chennai - 600030 • e-mail: chennai@cbspd.com

Printed at : Somya Printers, Delhi

PREFACE

Life is a continuous learning process. Human beings are born to learn and gain knowledge. Education is a means to acquire knowledge and skills that an individual desires to practise. Examinations are the means to evaluate the knowledge. Though no method of evaluation is without flaw, the process of standardization has resulted in a multiple choice system of examination. This system satisfies the basic qualities of a measuring instrument viz., validity, reliability and objectivity.

Recently, a number of books have been published about these examinations but the **best book still remains that which covers the maximum number of questions, which had been asked in that particular examination,** because the chance of repetition of these questions from so-called **"Question Bank"** remains very high. Recently, it has been observed that many **"Question Banks"** have overlapped. So, it is best to do a book which is complete and covers the **"Question Banks"** of maximum number of examinations. This book is being forwarded in this direction.

This book is designed as a supplement to the standard textbooks. It includes the **Referenced - MCQ's** (of previous years papers) of various PG Medical Entrance and Services Examinations **speciality-wise and Chapter-wise** arranged. The students while preparing the text or just before the examination can quickly go through this book. This will help in detecting the areas of weakness in understanding the text and thus, will improve the skills with multiple choice system of examination. It is a favourite book for **"Paper-setters".**

The importance of doing MCQ's alongwith text has increased tremendously because, recently, it has become a tendency to frame MCQ's usually not covered by the standard textbooks followed at undergraduate level. **"Quick Medical Text Review Series"** can be a useful adjuant to this book.

Beware of the **Fraudulent Books** available in the market, which covers a part of copied **'Question Bank'** from this book, and also, based on **'Constructed'** rather than **'Original'** Question Book. It is suggested not to waste time on these books. Every MCQ matters a lot in a highly competitive exams.

I request the readers not to forget to send their opinions, as also suggestions and contributions if any, about all aspects of this book. It will be of invaluable help in enhancing the utility of the book in future.

All suggestions are welcome and will be duly acknowledged in future editions.

— Editors

A book of the Readers, for the Readers, by the Readers

NOTE

The MCQ's of multiple response type (i.e. with **more than one correct answer** have been omitted in this Edition. Kindly refer to separate books **(PGI MD Entrance Exam & DNB Entrance Exam.** Part-I) by the same author and Publishers.

ADVICE

Read carefully the suggestions in the beginning of this book.

Prepare text from books suggested in the beginning and go through **Referenced MCQ's** of this book. Don't waste time in inexperienced, **incomplete and fraudulent courses books for PG Medical Entrance Examinations.**

ABOUT THE BOOK

This book has been compiled with the main aim to help the students to **quickly revise the Chapter-wise up-to-date referenced question** asked in various entrance examinations (Years indicated in the brackets).

Quick Medical Examinations Review Series contains Speciality-wise 45,000 MCQ's based on up-to-date papers from 1978 onwards.

The important examinations covered in this book (with code word in the bracket) are :

	Examinations	*Code used*
(A)	***All India level***	
1.	All India Postgraduate Entrance Examination	(AI)
2.	AIIMS MD Entrance Examination	(AIIMS)
3.	PGI MD Entrance Examination	(PGI)
4.	Combined Medical Services Examination by UPSC	(UPSC)
5.	Civil Services Entrance Examination, Part-I (Medicine)	(CS)
6.	Army Medical Corps Entrance Examination	(AMC)
7.	Diplomate of National Board Entrance Examination	(DNB)
8.	NIMHANS PG Entrance Examination	(NIMHANS)
9.	Sanjay Gandhi PG Institute Entrance Examination	(SGPGI)
10.	CIP Ranchi PG Entrance Examination	(CIP)
11.	Manipal Academy of Higher Education PG Entrance Examination	(Manipal/MAHE)
12.	Sree Chitra Tirunal Institute for Medical Science & Technology	(SCTIMST)
13.	Command Hospital, Bangalore	(CH)
14.	Bhabha Atomic Research Centre	(BARC)
15.	Institute of Aerospace Medicine	(IAM)
(B)	***State level***	
16.	Delhi MD Entrance Examination	(Delhi)
17.	Bihar MD Entrance Examination	(Bihar)
18.	JIPMER PG Entrance Examination	(JIPMER)
19.	CMC PG Entrance Examination	(CMC)
20.	Rohtak PG Entrance Examination	(Rohtak)
21.	MP State PG Entrance Examination	(MP)
22.	AP State MD Entrance Examination	(AP)
23.	TN State MD Entrance Examination	(TN)
24.	Karnataka Postgraduate Medical Entrance Examination	(Karnataka)
25.	Maharashtra PG Entrance Examination	(Maharashtra)
26.	Kerala State MD Entrance Examination	(Kerala)
27.	Rajasthan Postgraduate Entrance Examination	(Rajasthan)
28.	PG Entrance Examination, Varanasi	(BHU)
29.	Burdwan University	(BU)
30.	Combined Entrance Examination for PG Courses, U.P.	(UP)
31.	Punjab State PG Entrance Examination	(Punjab)
32.	Aligarh Muslim University PG Entrance Examination	(AMU)
33.	Nizam's Institute Entrance Examination, Hyderabad	(Nizam's)
34.	Postgraduate Admission Test, Orissa	(Orissa)
35.	Calcutta University Public Service Commission	(CUPSC)
36.	TN Public Service Commission	(TNPSC)
37.	Calcutta PG Entrance Examination	(Calcutta)
(C)	***Foreign***	
	PLAB, FCGP, GMC, FLEX, USMLE, MRCP, FRCS, MRCOG, etc.	

Sources of Errors (Radiology)

Example 1 : **Multiple calcifications in chest may be seen in :** **Karnataka 1988**

A. Histoplasmosis
B. Tropical eosinophilia
C. Tuberculosis
D. Measles

Answer : Both (A) and (C). **A wrongly framed** question

Example 2 : **Radiological feature of raised intracranial pressure in adults is :** **Karnataka 1989, 91, 93**

A. Expansion of sella turcica
B. Enlarged internal auditory meatus
C. Erosion of clinoid process
D. Gaping of sagittal sutures

Answer : Both (A) & (C) **A wrongly framed question.**

Example 3 : **String sign is seen in :** **Delhi 1983, Rohtak 1987**

A. Crohn's disease
B. Ileocaecal TB
C. Idiopathic hypertrophic pyloric stenosis
D. Irritable bowel syndrome

Answer : (A,B,C). Question should have contained **except,** then answer would have been choice (D)

Example 4 : **X-ray films are least sensitive to which coloured light :** **AIIMS 1986**

A. Violet
B. Blue
C. Yellow
D. Green

Answer : Choice (D) but if "red" would have been in the choices, it should have been the answer

Example 5 : **The following anticancer drug is cardiotoxic :** **AIIMS 1986, 89**

A. Cycloserine
B. Bleomycin
C. Adriamycin
D. Daunorubicin

Answer : (C) & (D) (Harrison's Principles of Internal Medicine)

Bleomycin may also cause acute (non-ischemic) chest pain.

Advice

Questions with inaccurate language (structuring) or wrong choices should better be left unattempted.

IMPORTANT RADIOLOGY TEXT FOR MCQ'S

CNS	Anatomy and Diseases of skull and spine, Anatomy and Diseases of Brain (Calcification, Tumours, Haematomas, Demyelinating lesions, Cystic lesions etc.)
Chest	Lung (Consolidation, Cavitating lesions, Collapse, Calcification), Mediastinum (Masses), Pleura (Pneumothorax, Haemo/ Hydrothorax); Diaphragm (Elevated, defects, Gas under it), Disorders (Defects) of chest wall, injuries, Breast (Calcification, mass, Mamography)
CVS	Heart (Enlargement of different chambers, Pericardial calcification and effusion, Infarction), Anomalous vasculature, Special appearances
GIT	Oesophagus (Achalasia, Carcinoma), Stomach and Duodenum (Ulcer Carcinoma, Duodenal atresia), Jejunum, Ileum (Atresia), Large bowel (Diverticulosis Carcinoma, Megacolon), Intestinal obstruction, Crohn's, Ulcerative colitis, T.B., Amoebiasis, Liver (Enlargement, Masses), Gall bladder (Stones, Calcification), Pancreas (Pancreatitis, Tumours). Spleen (Rupture, Masses)
Urogenital System	Peritoneum (Ascites), Polycystic/Horseshoe kidney, Hydronephrosis, TB, Flea beaten, White enlarged, Atrophy, Calculi, Bladder (Calculi, Diverticuli, Carcinoma), Adrenal (Calcification, Tumours), Male Genital Tract (Testicular masses, Tumours, Calcification), Female Genital Tract (Ovarian, Uterine and Cervix, Infertility, Estimation of foetal maturity), Pregnancy (foetal maturity)
Musculoskeletal System	Anatomy of bone, Estimation of age, Epiphyseal fusion, Osteolytic, Osteosclerotic secondaries, Tumours, Changes in Important Systemic Diseases, Congenital & Developmental disorders, Fractures.
Radiotherapy	Radioisotopes (common ones, half lives, specific indication), Effects of radiations, Specific uses, Techniques and Adverse effects
Radio Imaging	Diagnostic views (of skull, chest, Paranasal sinuses, Effusions), Techniques (Contrast medias used esp. in Carotid angiography, Bronchography, I.V.P. Myelography etc.), CT Scan, MRI
Miscellaneous	Named Views/Signs/Appearances; Factual data

IMPORTANT TIPS OF RADIOLOGY

Read	
* Causes of Periosteal new bone formation	Sutton's **Textbook of Radiology & Imaging**
* D/D of Aseptic bone necrosis	Sutton's **Textbook of Radiology & Imaging**
* Laboratory findings in Metabolic diseases	Sutton's **Textbook of Radiology & Imaging**
* Sites of Avulsion fracture & muscle origin	Sutton's **Textbook of Radiology & Imaging**
* D/D of Kerley Lines	Sutton's **Textbook of Radiology & Imaging**
* Fluid levels on a chest radiograph	Sutton's **Textbook of Radiology & Imaging**
* Anatomical locations of mediastinal masses	Sutton's **Textbook of Radiology & Imaging**
* Causes of calcification in mediastinum masses	Sutton's **Textbook of Radiology & Imaging**
* Intravascular contrast media	Sutton's **Textbook of Radiology & Imaging**
* Causes of small bowel fluid levels	Sutton's **Textbook of Radiology & Imaging**
* Small bowel vs large bowel dilatation	Sutton's **Textbook of Radiology & Imaging**
* D/D of abdomen calcification	Sutton's **Textbook of Radiology & Imaging**
* Causes of splenomegaly	Sutton's **Textbook of Radiology & Imaging**
* Obstetrics ultrasound	Sutton's **Textbook of Radiology & Imaging**
* Normal intracranial calcifications	Sutton's **Textbook of Radiology & Imaging**
* Pathological intracranial calcifications	Sutton's **Textbook of Radiology & Imaging**
* Causes of calcification of basal ganglia	Sutton's **Textbook of Radiology & Imaging**
* About mediastinal masses	Bhatia's **Quick Medical Text Review Series, Radiology**
* About Sutural and Skull thickness abnormalities	Bhatia's **Quick Medical Text Review Series, Radiology**
* About Roentgen signs in CVS	Bhatia's **Quick Medical Text Review Series, Radiology**
* About Radioisotopes	Tables in Bhatia's **Quick Medical Text Review Series, Radiology**
* About important views and appearances in different diseases	Bhatia's **Quick Medical Text Review Series, Radiology**
* About Radiation hazards	Tables in Bhatia's **Quick Medical Text Review Series, Radiology**
* About causes of Rib notching	Sutton's **Radiology and Imaging**, page 344.or Bhatia's **Quick Medical Text Review Series, Radiology**

CONTENTS

PSYCHIATRIC NURSING

(Dr. M.S. Bhatia, M.D., Dip. W.P.A)

About this book

- **This book : a must for :**
  - All Nursing Paramedical Students
  - Psychiatric Nursing
- This new book is specifically written for easy grasping of Psychiatry in a clearent, pointwise, simple and easy understandable language and is exclusively based on the examination and practice oriented pattern.
- Each chapter is followed by important Facts and Review Questions.
- A section on the general principles of psychiatry with a special emphasis on the **historical aspects,** aetiology, sympto-matology, psychiatric examination and **Glossary** has been included.
- An updated section on psychiatric treatment —including newer advances has been added.
- **Important topics** on Indian Psychiatry (Contributions of various Psychiatrists, Epidemiology of various disorders, manpower, National Mental Health Programme of India, Forensic Psychiatry etc.) have been explained.
- An important list of appendices include list of Psychotropic Drugs (Alphabetically, trade name wise, main indications, dosages and preparations) and a list of psychological tests commonly used in India.
- This concised textbook aimed at important **comprehensive theoretical** and **practical skills** in psychiatry and allied disciplines.

CBS Publishers & Distributors Pvt. Ltd.

NEW DELHI • BANGALORE • PUNE • CHENNAI • COCHIN (INDIA)

1

IMPORTANT TEXT OF CNS

SKULL

HYPERDENSE LESIONS

Increased density of falx

1. Subarachnoid hemorrhage
2. Interhemispheric subdural hematoma
3. Diffuse cerebral edema (=increased density relative to low density brain).
4. Dural calcifications (hypercalcemia from chronic renal failure, basal cell nevus syndrome, hyperparathyroidism).
5. Normal falx (can be normal in pediatric population).

Intracranial calcifications

Mnemonic : "PINEAL"
Physioligic
Infection
Neoplasm
Endocrine
Embryologic
Atriovenous
Leftover Lesions

A. *Physiologic* intracranial calcifications:

Pineal gland (10 years of age), choroid plexus (>3 years of age), habenular commissure (>10 years of age), petroclinoid ligament(>5 years of age), falx/tentorium (>3 years of age).

B. *Infection:*

Torch(toxoplasmosis, rubella, CMV, herpes), healed abscess, hydrated cyst, tuberculoma, cysticerosis mnemonic :

CMV calcifications are circumventricular (CV=CV)

Toxoplasma classifications are intraparenchymal (T=T)

C. *Neoplasm :*

Craniopharyngioma (40-80%), oligodendroglioma (50-70%) chordoma (25-40%), choroids plexus papilloma (10%), meningioma (20%), pituitary adenoma (3-5%), pinealoma (10-20%), dermoid (20%), lipoma of corpus callosum, ependymoma (50%), astrocytoma (15%), radiotherapy.

D. *Endocrine :*

Hyperparathyroidism, hypervitaminosis-D, hypoparathyroidism, pseudohypoparathyroidism, CO poisoning, lead poisoning.

E. *Embryologic :*

Neurocutaneous syndromes (tuberous sclerosis, Sturge-Weber, Neurofibromatosis), Fahr disease, Cockayne syndrome, basal cell nevus syndrome

F. *Arteriovenous :*

Atherosclerosis, aneurysm, AVM, hemangioma, subdural hematoma

G. *Leftover Lesions:*

Lipoma, lipoid proteinosis, lissencephaly

Basal ganglia calcification

A. *Physiologic with aging*

B. *Metabolic*
1. Hypoparathyroidism + Pseudohypoparathyroidism (60%)
2. Wilson disease
3. Fahr disease
4. Cockayne syndrome
5. Down's syndrome

C. *Trauma*
1. Childhood leukemia following methotrexate therapy
2. Post radiation
3. Birth anoxia

D. *Drugs*
1. Carbon monoxide poisoning
2. Lead intoxication

E. *Infection*
   1. Toxoplasmosis
   2. AIDS

Periventricular calcifications in a child

1. Tuberous sclerosis
2. Congenital infection : CMV, toxoplasmosis

INCIDENCE OF BRAIN TUMORS

= 9% of all primary neoplasms; account for 1.2% of autopsied deaths

In all Age groups		*In pediatric age group*	
Glioma	34%	Astrocytoma	50%
Meningioma	17%	Medulloblastoma	15%
Metastasis	12%	Ependymoma	10%
Pituitary adenoma	6%	Craniopharyngioma	6%
Neurinoma	4%	Choroid plexus papilloma	2%
Sarcoma	3%		
Granuloma	3%		
Craniopharyngioma	2%		

Tumors possibly presenting at birth :

1. Teratoma
2. Choroid plexus papilloma
3. Ependymoma
4. Craniopharyngioma
5. Astrocytoma
6. Medullablastoma

SUPRASELLAR MASS WITH CALCIFICATION :

A. *Curvilinear :*
   1. Giant carotid aneurysm
   2. Craniopharyngioma

B. *Granular :*
   1. Craniopharyngioma
   2. Meningioma
   3. Granuloma
   4. Dermoid cyst/teratoma
   5. Optic/hypothalamic glioma (rare)

MCQ's OF CNS

What is important in CNS

Anatomy amd Diseases of skull and spine, Anatomy and Diseases of Brain (Calcification, Tumours, Haematomas, Demyelinating lesions, Cystic lesions etc.)

1. Commonest cause of 'ring blush' in brain is : AIIMS 1982, 93

A. Glioblastoma B. Metastasis
C. Abscess D. Grade-II astrocytoma

2. After acoustic neuroma, the second commonest cerebellopontine angle tumor is : AMU 1985, 91

A. Trigeminal neuroma B. Epidermoid tumor
C. Glioma D. Medulloblastoma

3. Mastoid process is best seen on : AIIMS 1980, 85, 97

A. A base view B. AP laminography
C. Lateral oblique view D. Transorbital projection

4. Match the following: UPSC 1990

Calcification	Cerebral lesion
I. Rounded balls (Brain stones)	i. Struge Weber syndrome
II. Curvilinear	ii. Anurysm near sella tursica
III. Albl's ring	iii. Tuberous sclerosis
IV. Tramline calci- carotid artery	iv. Atheroma of fication

A. I (ii) II (iii) III (iv) IV (i)
B. I (iii) II (iv) III (ii) IV (i)
C. I (iv) II (iii) III (ii) IV (i)
D. I (i) II (ii) III (iii) IV (iv)

5. Fresh blood in CT Scan appears as : AI 1994; Rajasthan 2001

A. Hyperdense B. Isodense
C. Hypodense D. Any of the above

6. Best view for evaluating sella turcica is : AI 1994, 99

A. Lateral X-ray skull B. AP X-ray skull
C. Towne's view D. Open mouth

7. Procedure of choice in diagnosing empty sella syndrome is : AIIMS 1991, 98

A. Pneumoencephalography
B. Caldwell X-ray view
C. CT scan
D. MRI

8. Geographic lytic lesion in vault of skull with bevelled edges is : AIIMS 1995

A. Multiple myeloma
B. Eosinophilic granuloma
C. Hyperparathyroidism
D. Paget's disease

9. Ideal modality to diagnose hydrocephalus in a 1 month baby is : Rajasthan 1991; MP 1994

A. Plain X-ray B. Ultrasound
C. CT scan D. MRI

10. Cerebral calcification is a feature of : PGI 1987, 91, 97, 2002

A. Congenital syphilis
B. Cytomegalic inclusion disease
C. Alzheimer's syndrome
D. Fanconi's syndrome

11. Echoencephalography is most useful for detecting : PGI 1986, 89

A. Ventricular dilatation B. Midline shift
C. Epilepsy D. Vascular lesions

12. Craniotabes is seen in following except : PGI 1997

A. Fanconi syndrome B. Renal tubular acidosis
C. Rickets D. None of the above

13. Enhancement in MRI is basal ganglia & thalamus is seen in : PGI 2000, 2003

A. Rabies
B. Herpes simplex encephalitis
C. Lymphocytic choriomeningitis
D. Creutz Jacob's disease

Ans. 1. C 2. D 3. C 4. B 5. A 6. A 7. D 8. B 9. B 10. B
11. A 12. D 13. D

14. "Tear Drop" sign in CT scan is seen in : UP 1998, 2000

A. Blow out # of orbit B. # Zygoma
C. Maxillary sinus D. Posteriocranial fossa #

15. Investigation of choice for screening of proximal internal carotid artery stenosis is : AIIMS 2000

A. Doppler flow USG
B. CT substraction angiography
C. MRI
D. Angiography (DSA)

16. Sialogram is used to study : AI 1996

A. Salivary glands B. Lymph glands
C. Thyroid D. Pituitary

17. CSF on MRI scan appears : Delhi 2001

A. Hyperintense on T1 weighted image and hypointense on T2 weighted images.
B. Hypointense on T1 weighted image and hyperintense on T2 weighted images.
C. Hyperintense on T1 and T2 weighted images.
D. Hypointense on T1 and T2 weighted images.

18. Bracket calcification of skull X-ray is seen in : JIPMER 2002

A. Meningioma
B. Sturge- Weber's syndrome
C. Corpus callosum lipoma
D. Tuberous sclerosis

19. Unilateral orbital enlargement occurs in following except : DNB 1990

A. Neurofibromatosis
B. Carotico-cavernous fistula
C. Meningioma
D. Thyrotoxicosis
E. Rhabdomyosarcoma

20. The following cause lytic lesions in the skull vault : DNB 1990

A. Dystrophia mytonica
B. Albers-Shonberg disease
C. Craniometaphyseal dysplasia
D. Chordoma
E. Hand-Schuller-Christian disease

21. Investigation of choice in head injury is : UPSC 1984

A. X-ray skull B. CT Scan
C. MRI D. EEG

22. Basal ganglia calcification in hilar region is seen in : AI 1989

A. Wilson's disease B. Berry aneurysm
C. Cysticercosis D. Hemangioma

23. 'Intracranial 'C' shaped calcification is see in : AIIMS 1993

A. Pineal B. Habenular commisure
C. Falx D. Thalamus

24. 5th ventricle is : AIIMS 1984

A. Cavum vergae
B. Cavum septi pellucidi
C. Cavum veli interpositi
D. Colloid cyst

25. Causes of posterior soft tissues nasopharyngeal mass include all except : AMU 1986

A. Plasmacytoma
B. Choana atresia
C. Thornwaldt's cyst
D. Aneurysm of the carotid artery
E. Chordoma

26. Rain drop lesions in skull are classically seen in : DNB 1997

A. Osteomalacia B Multiple myeloma
C. Head injury D. CML

27. Punched out translucencies in the skull does not occur in one of the conditions given below : Delhi 1985

A. Multiple myeloma B. Metastatic deposits
C. Leukaemia D. Fluorosis

28. Thymus is usually small or absent in all of the following except : DNB 1990

A. Leukaemia B. Congenital rubella
C. Prematurity D. Di George syndrome
E. None of these

29. The metastatic lesions may be present as subarachnoid hemorrhage: AMU 1987

A. Seminoma B. Lymphoma
C. Malignant melanoma D. Reticulum cell sarcoma
E. Ovarian cystadenoma

30. Which of the following is not paired structure : DNB 1989

A. Anterior clinoid B. Internal cerebral vein
C. Cribriform plate D. Foramen of Monro
E. Precentral cerebellar vein

31. Convolutional markings in a child usually do not appear until----------- of age : AMU 1985

A. 3 months B. 6 months
C. 12 months D. 3 years
E. 12 years

32. Tram-line calcification is seen in : Delhi 1987

A. Ependymoma
B. Thrombosed cerebral vein
C. Meningioma
D. Sturge-Weber syndrome

Ans.										
	14. A	15. A	16. A	17. B	18. C	19. D	20. E	21. B	22. A	23. B
	24. B	25. B	26. B	27. D	28. A	29. C	30. E	31. D	32. D	

33. **True about maxillary sinusitis in X-ray PNS is : Rajasthan 1996**
A. If polyps are seen it suggests allergy.
B. Fluid level is seen.
C. If surrounding bone shows sclerosis it suggests infection.
D. Infective sinusitis is usually unilateral.

34. **Earliest sign of raised intracranial pressure in adults is : AI 1991, 96**
A. Erosion of anterior clinoid process
B. Erosion of posterior clinoid process
C. Enlargement of sella
D. Silver beaten appearance

35. **CT scan of a 60 years old male who had a fall presenting with confusion is most likely to reveal : Rajasthan 1991; UPSC 1994**
A. Cerebral atrophy
B. Glioma
C. Normal pressure hydrocephalus
D. Subdural haematoma

36. **Internal auditory canals of both sides are best visualized in : DNB 1991**
A. Occipitofrontal B. Sub-mento vertical
C. Lateral D. None of the above

37. **On usual CT scale of densities (-1000 to + 1000), brain tissue measures : AIIMS 1986, 89**
A. -10 to +10 B. 0 to +20
C. +10 to +30 D. +20 to +45
E. +50 to +100

38. **Which of the following is wrong regarding 'J' shaped sella : DNB 1989**
A. Normal variant in 30% of cases
B. Seen in optic glioma
C. Mucopolysaccharidoses
D. Low grade hydrocephalus

39. **Suprasellar calcification is seen in following except : Karnataka 1989; AIIMS 1985, 94; AI 1997; JIPMER 2002, 2006**
A. Craniopharyngioma B. Meningioma
C. Calcified pineal gland D. Pituitary adenoma

40. **Cerebral angiography is useful in demonstrating : AIIMS 1985**
A. Lesions of cerebral blood vessels and intracranial tumours
B. Scars and atrophic lesions of the brain
C. Chronic meningitis
D. Epilepsy

41. **CT scan in acute subdural hematoma shows : AIIMS 1998**
A. Biconvex hyperdense shadow
B. Concavoconvex hyperdense shadow
C. Biconvex hypodense shadow
D. Attenuated hypodense shadow

42. **'Bare Orbit' appearance of skull is seen in : DNB 1989**
A. Multiple myeloma B. Meningioma
C. Neurofibromatosis D. Craniopharyngioma

43. **Which is not true regarding medulloblastoma : PGI 1985; AI 1990**
A. Radio-resistant tumor
B. Highly radio-sensitive
C. Generally occurs in first decade
D. Commonly spreads through CSF

44. **Commonest calcified brain tumour is : Delhi 1987, 88; AIIMS 1986**
A. Craniopharyngioma B. Meningioma
C. Tuberculoma D. Medulloblastoma

45. **Which of the normal calcifications may be considered abnormal and suggestive of pseudohypoparathyroidism : AIIMS 1986, 90; PGI 1994**
A. Choroid plexuses B. Basilar ganglia
C. Pineal gland D. Petroclinoid ligament

46. **Premature filling of veins in cerebral angiography is a manifestation of : AMU 1985**
A. Trauma
B. Brain tumour
C. Arteriovenous malformation
D. Arterial occlusion

47. **X-ray changes in acromegaly are following except : Delhi 1997**
A. Lengthened terminal phalanx
B. Widened joint spaces
C. Obtuse angle of mandible
D. Premature osteoarthritis

48. **In tuberous sclerosis there is, except : AIIMS 1985**
A. Sclerosis of the distal phalanges.
B. An increased chance of hamartoma of the kidney.
C. An increased incidence of hepatoma.
D. An increased incidence of cardiac rhabdomyoma.
E. An increased incidence of cerebral glioma.

49. **The crescent sign seen in a brain scan commonly indicates a subdural hematoma. It may also be seen in : AMU 1987, 93**
A. Dural metastases B. Pachymeningitis
C. Both D. Neither

Ans. 33. D 34. B 35. D 36. A 37. D 38. A 39. D 40. A 41. B 42. C
43. A 44. A 45. B 46. C 47. A 48. C 49. C

50. The 'doughnut' sign on a brain scan usually suggests: DNB 1989

A. Abscess
B. Metastases
C. Glioblastoma
D. All of the above

51. Optic foramen enlargement on X-ray skull is suggestive of : JIPMER 1992

A. Meningioma
B. Optic N-glioma
C. Retinoblastoma
D. Carotico-cavernous fistula

52. Intracranial calcification in X-ray can be due to : TN 1993; Rajasthan 1998

A. Pineal calcification
B. Dural calcification
C. Cysticercosis
D. All of the above

53. Signs of increased intracranial tension in a child in a skull X-ray : AMU 1984, 90, 98

A. Separation of the sutures
B. Tense anterior fontanelle
C. Silver beaten appearance of the bones
D. All of the above

54. Which of the following is not true about CT scan in head injury : Delhi 1997

A. Subarachnoid haemorrhages increase in density over serial CT scans.
B. Extradural haematoma appears as biconvex shadow.
C. Subdural haematoma appears as crescent shadow.
D. Intracerebral contusion initially produces no CT signs or area of low attenuation.

55. Intracranial calcification is seen in all except: AIIMS 1983

A. Lipoma of corpus collosum
B. Medulloblastoma
C. Tuberculoma
D. Ependymoma
E. Neurofibromatosis

56. Which of the following brain tumors does not spread via CSF : AI 2004

A. Germ cell tumors
B. Medulloblastoma
C. CNS Lymphoma
D. Craniopharyngioma

57. Investigation of choice for acoustic neuroma : AIIMS 2008

A. CT without contrast
B. CT with contrast
C. MRI without contrast
D. MRI with contrast

58. All of the following is feature of temporal lobe epilepsy except : AI 2009

A. Atrophy of fomices
B. Atrophy of temporal lobe
C. Atrophy of hippocampus
D. Atrophy of mammillary body

59. Cerebral blood flow in asphyxiated infant is measured by : AIIMS 2009

A. EEG
B. Infrared spectroscopy
C. PET
D. Perfusion MRI

60. A 40 years old female presented with recurrent headaches. MRI showed extra axial, dural based and enhancing lesion. The most likely diagnosis is : Delhi 2009

A. Meaningioma
B. Glioma
C. Schwannoma
D. Pituitary adenoma

Ans. 50. D 51. B 52. D 53. D 54. A 55. B 56. D 57. D 58. B 59. B 60. A

EXPLANATIONS OF CNS

1. Ans.— C. Abscess
2. Ans.— D. Medulloblastoma
3. Ans.— C. Lateral oblique view
4. Ans.— B. I (iii) II (iv) III (ii) IV (i)
5. Ans.— A. Hyperdense
6. Ans.— A. Lateral X-ray skull

   Best used is Cone's view.
7. Ans.— D. MRI
8. Ans.— B. Eosinophilic granuloma
9. Ans.— B. Ultra sound
10. Ans.— B. Cytomegalic inclusion disease
11. Ans.— A. Ventricular dilatation
12. Ans.— D. None of the above
13. Ans.— D. Creutz Jacob's disease
14. Ans.— A. Blow out # of orbit
15. Ans.— A. Doppler flow USG
16. Ans.— A. Salivary glands
17. Ans.— B. Hypointense on T1 weighted image and hyperintense on T2 weighted image.
18. Ans.— C. Corpus callosum lipoma
19. Ans.— D. Thyrotoxicosis
20. Ans.— E. Hand-Schuller-Christian disease

    Osteolytic lesion of skull are seen in :-

    Normal (Venous lake, Pacchionian granulations or due to parietal foraminae), Trauma (Surgical burr hole, leptomeningeal cyst), Infection (osteomyelitis, hydatid, TB, Syphilis), Congenital (epidermoid/desmoid, neuro-fibromatosis (asterion defect), meningo-encephalocele, fibrous dysplasia, osteoporosis circumscripta of Paget's disease), Benign tumour (haemangioma, brown tumor, eosinophilic granuloma) and Malignant tumor (solitary/multiple metastasis, multiple myeloma, leukemia, neuroblastoma).
21. Ans.— B. CT Scan
22. Ans.— A. Wilson's disease
23. Ans.— B. Habenular commisure
24. Ans.— B. Cavum septi pellucidi
25. Ans.— B. Choana atresia
26. Ans.— B Multiple myeloma
27. Ans.— D. Fluorosis
28. Ans.— A. Leukaemia
29. Ans.— C. Malignant melanoma
30. Ans.— E. Precentral cerebellar vein
31. Ans.— D. 3 years
32. Ans.— D. Sturge-Weber syndrome
33. Ans.— D. Infective sinusitis is usually unilateral
34. Ans.— B. Erosion of posterior clinoid process
35. Ans.— D. Subdural haematoma
36. Ans.— A. Occipitofrontal
37. Ans.— D. +20 to +45
38. Ans.— A. Normal variant in 30% of cases
39. Ans.— D. Pituitary adenoma

    Craniopharyngioma shows calcification in 70% cases, and is commonest cause. Meningioma shows calcification in 10% and Glioma in 7% cases.
40. Ans.— A. Lesions of cerebral blood vessels and intracranial tumours

    Cerebral angiography is useful in cerebral aneurysms, SAH, angiomas or vascular malformation, thrombotic or embolic occlusion.
41. Ans.— B. Concavoconvex hyperdense shadow
42. Ans.— C. Neurofibromatosis
43. Ans.— A. Radio-resistant tumor

    Pneumoperitoneum may be seen in trauma (penetrating or blunt injuries), spontaneous causes (peptic or bowel perforation, toxic megacolon) and other female genital tract lesions and pneumatosis intestinalis.
44. Ans.— A. Craniopharyngioma

45. Ans.— B. Basilar ganglia

46. Ans.— C. Arteriovenous malformation

47. Ans.— A. Lengthened terminal phalanx

48. Ans.— C. An increased incidence of hepatoma

49. Ans.— C. Both

50. Ans.— D. All of the above

51. Ans.— B. Optic N-glioma

52. Ans.— D. All of the above

Intracranial calcification is seen Mnemonic "PINEAL" Physiological (pineal gland above 10 years of age, choroid plexus above 3 years of age, habenular commissure above 10 years of age, petroclinoid ligament above 5 years of age and falx/tentorium above 3 years of age), Infection (TORCH, healed abscess, TB, cysticercosis, hydatidosis), Neoplasm Cranio-pharyngioma (40-80%), oligo-dendroglioma (50-70%), Chordoma (25-40%), Choroid plexus papilloma (10%), Meningioma (20%), Pituitary adenoma (3-5%), Pinealoma (10-20%), dermoid (20%), lipoma of corpus callosum, ependymoma (50%), astrocytoma (15%), radiotherapy, Endocrine, (hyperpara-thyroidsm, hypervitaminosis-D, hypo-parathyroidism, pseudo-hypopara-thyroidism, CO poisoning, lead poison-ing), Embryonic (Neurocutaneous syn-dromes tuberous- sclerosis, Sturge Weber, neuro-fibromatosis), Fahr's disease, Cockayne syndrome), Arteriovenous (atherosclero-sis, haematoma), Leftover (Lipoma, lipoid proteinosis, lissen-cephaly).

53. Ans.— D. All of the above

Chronic raised intracranial tension (ICT) may lead to "Silver beaten appearance" whereas in adults, erosion of posterior clinoid process is the earliest sign of raised ICT.

54. Ans.— A. Subarachnoid haemorrhages increase in density over serial CT scans.

55. Ans.— B. Medulloblastoma

56. Ans.— D. Craniopharyngioma

57. Ans.— D MR with contrast

58. Ans.— B. Atrophy of temporal lobe

Classical features include :

* Small hippocampus with increased signal on T2-weighted sequences
* Small temporal lobe
* Enlarged temporal horn

59. Ans.— B. Infrared spectroscopy

60. Ans.— A. Meaningioma

2

IMPORTANT TEXT OF CHEST

A. Coin Shaped (Solitary Cricrumscribed Nodules)

* Granulomas-Tuberculosis, Histoplasmosis, Coccidiodomycosis
* Cyst-bronchial, Hydatid
* Bronchial Adenoma
* Hamartomas
* Bronchogenic carcinoma
* Metastatic Nodule
* Chest wall Lesions-Mesothelioma or Fibroma of Pleura
* Others—Subpleural lymph nodes, Pneumonia, A V Fistula, Anthracosis, silicosis, Infarct, Lung abscesses.

B. Disseminated multiple pulmonary opacities (Miliary Mottling)

* Infections — Miliary TB, Bronchopneumonia, Brucellosis, Histoplasmosis, Coccidiodomycosis, Blastomycosis.
* Inhalations — Pneumoconiosis, Berylliosis, Iodisted Oil (bronchochography), Mineral Oil (nose drops), Aspiration.
* Caridovascular — Heamosiderosis, Pulmonary Oedema, Multiple Pulmonary infarcts, Fat emboli.
* Allergic — Loeffer's syndrome, Asthma, Ascarasis.
* Bronchial — Excessive bronchiectesis, Mucoviscidosis.
* Neoplastic — Alveoler cell carcinoma of bronchus.
* Reticulosis — Lymphadenoma. Lymphoma, Leukaemia, Polycythemia.
* Others — Sarcoidosis, Rheumatoid arthritis, Hyaline membrane disease, Interstitial fibrosis, Honey-comb lung.

C. Causes of Hypertranslucency

	Unilateral	*Bilateral*
Chestwall :	Mastectomy, Polio, Scoliosis	* Diffuse obstructive emphysema.
Congenital :	Absence of pectoral muscle	* Senile emphysema
Pulmonary :	Emphysema artery hypoplasia	* Bronchial asthma
	bullae : Main pulmonary artery hypoplasia	* Bullae
Pleura :	Pneumothorax, contralateral pleural	* Bilateral Pneumothorax
	Effusion or pleural thickening	* Massive embolism
		* Primary pulmonary hypertension
		* Congenital heart disease—Tetralogy of Fallot, Ebstein's anomaly, Pulmonary atresia.

D. Causes of Hilar Enlargement

Unilateral	*Bilateral*
* Tuberculosis	* Tuberculosis
* Bronchogenic carcinoma	* Sarcoidosis
* Metastatic adenopathy	* Fungal infection

* Sarcoidosis	* Lymphoma
* Fungal disease	* Pneumoconiosis
* Mediastinal masses	* Metastatic malignancy
* Lymphnode hyperplasia	* Erythema nodosum
* Others - Lymphatic leukaemia	* Others - Leukaemia
Pulmonary stenosis	acute massive pulmonary embolism

E. Causes of Cavitation in Chest

Cavity (containing air or fluid)	*Solid Mass within a cavity*
* Abscess	* Aspergillosis
* Bronchogenic carcinoma	* Blood clot in cavity
* Tuberculosis	* Breaking down neoplasm
* Mycotic cavitation	* Complicated hydatid cyst

F. Causes of Calcification in Chest

* Chest wall — Costal cartilages, Healing rib fractures, Tubercular glands, Cysticerci, breast tumour, Guinea worm, Osteomas, Chondromas
* Tracheobronchi — Senile
* Pleura — Plaques following T.B., Emphysema, Pneumoconiosis, Hemothorax
* Mediastinal — Lymphadenopathy (T.B., Sarcoid, Pneumoconiosis), Tumours (thyroid adenoma, aneurysm, dermoid cyst)
* Lungs — Infections (T.B., Abscess , Fabrotic scars, Fungal infections), Vascular (hematoma, AV aneurysm), tumours (Hamartoma, Secondaries), Unknown (Broncholiths, Mitral stenosis)
* Heart — Valves, Pericardium, Aortic arch (atherosclerosis, Syphilis), Left atrium (In MS), Coronary arteries, Patent ductus

G. Causes of Rib Notching

* Idiopathic
* Vascular — Coarctation of aorta, Taussig-Blalock operation, Obstructive artheritis, Pulmonary oligemia, (Pulmonary stenosis, Fallot's Tetralogy, Ebstein's anomaly), Venous (SVC or IVC obstruction), A V fistulae
* Neurofibromatosis

METASTASIS OF LUNG

Pulmonary metastasis occur in 30% of all malignancies; mostly hematogenous
Age : > 50 years (in 87%)
Frequency :

	Origin of pulmonary metastasis		*Probability of pulmonary metastasis*	
1.	Breast	22%	Kidney	75%
2.	Kidney	11%	Osteosarcoma	75%
3.	Head and Neck	10%	Choriocarcinoma	75%
4.	Colorectal	9%	Thyroid	65%
5.	Uterus	6%	Melanoma	60%
6.	Pancreas	5%	Breast	55%
7.	Ovary	5%	Prostate	40%
8.	Prostate	4%	Head and Neck	30%
9.	Stomach	4%	Esophagus	20%

MCQ's OF CHEST

What is important in Chest

Lung (Consolidation, Cavitating lesions, Collapse, Calcification), Mediastinum (Masses), Pleura (Pneumothorax, Haemo/Hydrothorax); Diaphragm (Elevated, defects, Gas under it), Disorders (Defects) of chest wall, injuries, Breast (Calcification, mass)

1. An elevated right hemidiaphragm following abdominal trauma should suggest: AIIMS 1983, 90, 97
A. Rupture of liver
B. Rupture of diaphragm
C. Right lower lobe atelectasis
D. Subpleural fluid

2. On serial chest film a nodule with tumour doubling time of over one year increase the probability that the lesion is : AMU 1986, 95
A. Cystic
B. Malignant
C. Benign
D. Inflammatory

3. Dilatation of upper lobe vein is a reliable sign of : AIIMS 1985, 89, 94
A. Hilar Tumour
B. Emphysema
C. Pulmonary hypertension
D. Cardiac decompensation

4. Chylothorax is associated with all except : DNB 1990, 97
A. Whipple's disease
B. Hodgkin's disease
C. Pulmonary lymphangiomyomatosis
D. Blunt chest trauma
E. Lymphangitis carcinomatosis

5. Water lilly appearance in chest X-ray is suggestive of : PGI 1982; AI 1994
A. Bronchiectasis
B. Broncheopleural fistula
C. Hydatid cyst
D. Sequestration cyst of lung

6. In a child, pneumatocele formation is seen in all except: AIIMS 1985; AI 1998
A. Escherichia coli pneumonia
B. Streptococcal pneumonia
C. Hydrocarbon ingestion
D. Goodpasture's syndrome
E. Tuberculosis

7. Hypertrophic pulmonary osteoarthropathy occurs with following except: AMU 1986, 91, 95
A. Fibrosing alveolitis
B. Pleural fibroma
C. Squamous carcinoma of the bronchus
D. Goodpasture's syndrome

8. Increased radiolucency of one sided hemithorax may be caused by following except : AIIMS 1986; AI 1990
A. Expiratory films
B. Pneumothorax
C. Patient rotation
D. Obstructive emphysema

9. Normal pulmonary arterial pressure (mmHg) in systole is : PGI 1984, 89
A. 10 - 12
B. 12 - 16
C. 16 - 20
D. 25 - 30
E. 30 - 35

10. Calcification in pulmonary metastasis may be found most often in: PGI 1986, 89
A. Osteosarcoma
B. Papillary carcinoma thyroid
C. Chondrosarcoma
D. Ovarian cystadenoma
E. Carcinoma of breast

11. Local tracheal displacement in the neck is most commonly due to : PGI 1984, 94
A. Marked Pleural effusion
B. Atelectesis
C. Enlarged thyroid
D. Thyroiditis
E. Cyst

Ans. 1. B 2. C 3. D 4. A 5. C 6. D 7. D 8. A 9. D 10. A 11. C

12. The most common underlying scar for scar carcinoma in lungs is: **Delhi 1984**
A. Infarct B. Granuloma
C. Tuberculoma D. Fibrotic scar

13. Typical carcinoid in lungs presents as : **AIIMS 1986**
A. Lobar collapse
B. Obstructive pneumonitis
C. Hilar mass
D. Any of the above

14. Pneumothorax is not a feature in: **Karnataka 1989**
A. Honeycomb lungs B. Bronchiectasis
C. Tuberculosis D. Emphysema

15. Round pneumonias occur in : **Delhi 1985**
A. Children B. Adult males
C. Adult females D. Elderly

16. Cavitating pulmonary metastasis are usually from: **Delhi 1983**
A. Testes B. Colon
C. Kidneys D. Cervix

17. The following are the cardiophrenic angle masses except: **AMU 1987**
A. Pericardial cyst
B. Diaphgragmatic hernia through foramen of Morgagni
C. Epicardial nodes
D. Bronchogenic cyst

18. Fibrosing mediastinitis may result due to: **AIIMS 1985.**
A. Tuberculosis B. Histoplasmosis
C. Iatrogenic D. Any of the above

19. Primary lung cancer is unlikely if a solitary pulmonary nodule: **DNB 1990**
A. Has well-defined margins
B. Has spiculated margins
C. Contains pleural tag
D. There is no growth for at least 2 years

20. Pancoast tumour is more commonly seen in ——— type: **Delhi 1985**
A. Squamous B. Columnar
C. Adeno D. Pseudostratified

21. The intensity of colour in Doppler is determined by: **PGI 1998**
A. Direction of flow
B. Velocity of flow
C. Strength of returning echo
D. Duration of flow

22. Kerley's A& B lines are: **DNB 1990; AIIMS 1997**
A. Thickened interlobular septa
B. Linear atelectatic lung shadow
C. Vascular shadow
D. Lymphatic shadow

23. Pulmonary embolism is best diagnosed by : **AI 1996**
A. CT Scan
B. Ventilation-perfusion scan
C. X-ray Chest
D. Pulmonary function

24. Following trauma to the chest, an increasing hemothorax suggest that bleeding source is : **AIIMS 1984**
A. From pulmonary vessel
B. Unrelated to trauma
C. From the lung
D. Not from the lung

25. The best view of the chest to show minimal sub-pulmonary effusion is : **TN 1988**
A. PA view B. AP view
C. Lateral decubitus view D. Oblique view

26. Middle lobe collapse may be demonstrated to best advantage on the : **Delhi 1981; AIIMS 1985**
A. Frontal projection B. Lateral projection
C. Lordotic projection D. Overexposed view

27. A pulmonary consolidation in a patient with asthma is frequently due to : **PGI 1982, 83**
A. Aspergillosis B. Fibrosis
C. Tuberculosis D. Cryptococcosis

28. One of the primary differential points between pulmonary embolism and infarction is : **AMU 1984**
A. Clear lung fields B. Diaphragmatic change
C. Pleural fluid D. Hilar change

29. Persistent bilateral pulmonary change associated with acute renal failure occur in except: **AIIMS 1981**
A. Churge-Strauss syndrome
B. Goodpasture's syndrome
C. Wegener's granulomatosis
D. Acute pyelonephritis
E. Systemic lupus erythematosis

30. Pneumothorax is best demonstrated by taking a radiograph, with the patient in: **AIIMS 1983**
A. Inspiration B. Expiration
C. Full inspiration D. Full expiration
E. Supine

Ans.									
12. A	13. D	14. A	15. A	16. D	17. D	18. D	19. D	20. A	21. C
22. A	23. B	24. D	25. C	26. C	27. A	28. A	29. D	30. D	

31. During angiocardiography, accidental injection of contrast into the myocardium is : PGI 1982

A. Usually fatal
B. Markedly well tolerated
C. A common cause of ventricular fibrillation
D. Always followed by severe myocardial damage

32. The cause of single coin shadow in the lung with calcification in the center is : AIIMS 1986

A. Epidermoid carcinoma B. Adeno carcinoma
C. Melanoma D. Oat cell tumour

33. Oligaemic lung fields are seen in all of the following except: DNB 1989

A. Tetralogy of Fallot
B. Anomalous venus drainage
C. Tricuspid stenosis
D. Atrial septal defects

34. Sign of greatest value in diagnosis of pulmonary emphysema is : Orissa 1991; Rajasthan 1994

A. Hyperlucency
B. Hyperation
C. Change in calibre of arteries
D. Diaphragm depression

35. Most direct and reliable roentgen sign of lobar collapse is : BHU 1986

A. Air bronchogram
B. Displacement of interlobar septum
C. Mediastinal shift
D. Radio density

36. Primary importance of air bronchogram is to localise intrathoracic lesion as being : BHU 1986

A. Pneumonitis B. Atelectasis
C. Intrapulmonary D. Extrapulmonary

37. The lordotic view is valuable in confirming the presence of lesion in the lung apex and also in the : Delhi 1985

A. Posterior mediastinum
B. Lingular segment
C. Posterior basal segment
D. Hilum

38. The expiratory film is valuable in detecting a small pneumothorax because: Delhi 1984

A. Pleural pressure is fixed
B. Pleural pressure is diminished
C. Intra-pulmonary pressure is diminished
D. Intrapulmonary pressure is increased

39. Childhood tuberculosis is most often characterized by: AIIMS 1983

A. Pleural effusion
B. Infiltrate and nodal enlargement
C. Hilar enlargement and pleural fluid
D. Cavity lesions and hilar adenopathy

40. Bilateral calcification in lungs can occur in all except: BHU 1986; Karnataka 1987; AI 1989; MAHE 1994

A. Friedlanders pneumonia
B. Coccidiodomycosis
C. Histoplasmosis
D. Pulmonary tuberculosis

41. Causes of a cavitating lesion in the chest radiograph are except: AIIMS 1983

A. Harmartoma
B. Pulmonary infarction
C. Squamous carcinoma of the bronchus
D. Caplan's syndrome
E. Haematoma

42. Most frequent finding following a fracture of the trachea or bronchus is : AIIMS 1982

A. Pneumothorax B. Interstitial air
C. Deviation of trachea D. Pleural fluid

43. The nodular pattern often seen in the lungs following renal transplantation is thought to be due to : PGI 1987

A. Fungus B. Infarcts
C. Cytomegalovirus D. Autoimmune reaction

44. Most reliable sign of diaphragmatic paralysis: AIIMS 1987

A. Positive sniff test B. Unequal movement
C. Elevated diaphgragm D. Mediastinal shift

45. Pneumography is a method of examination for peritoneal or retroperitoneal structure. Gas used as contrast agent in this examination is : PGI 1982

A. Oxygen B. Nitrogen
C. Carbon dioxide D. Any of the above

46. Origin of Pulmonary metastasis is maximum from : AIIMS 1984, 87

A. Kidney B. Head and Neck
C. Ovary D. Breast

47. Ossific nodules in the lungs have been observed in: AIIMS 1984

A. Constructive pericarditis
B. Left atrial myxoma
C. Mitral stenosis
D. All of the above

Ans. 31. B 32. A 33. D 34. C 35. B 36. C 37. B 38. C 39. B 40. A 41. A 42. B 43. C 44. D 45. C 46. D 47. D

48. **Calcification can occur in pulmonary metastasis from the following except in : Bihar 1986**
A. Carcinoma of the pancreas
B. Carcinoma of the breast
C. Adenocarcinoma of the thyroid
D. Squamous cell carcinoma
E. Papillary cystadenoma carcinoma of the ovary

49. **Progressive massive fibrosis can occur in: AIIMS 1983**
A. Bagassosis B. Berylliosis
C. Silicosis D. Stannosis

50. **Fluoroscopy is indicated in the following: AIIMS 1981**
A. Chronic pulmonary tuberculosis
B. Early pulmonary tuberculosis
C. Acute miliary tuberculosis
D. In patient with specific complaints referable to chest

51. **The most common cause of spontaneous pneumothorax is: AMU 1986**
A. Tuberculosis
B. Bronchial adenoma
C. Bronchogenic carcinoma
D. Rupture of a subpleural bleb

52. **The following may result in miliary shadows on chest X-ray except: AMU 1986**
A. Sarcoidosis
B. Mitral Stenosis
C. Pneumoconiosis
D. Staphylococcal pneumonia

53. **The most common malignant tumour of the lung in smokers is: AI 1990; UPSC 1992**
A. Fibrosarcoma
B. Adenocarcinoma
C. Leiomyosarcoma
D. Squamous cell carcinoma

54. **Smoking causes ——— emphysema : Rajasthan 1998**
A. Panacinar B. Centriacinar
C. Irregular D. Rare septal

55. **One of the following causes mediastinal enlargement: AI 1995**
A. Diffused histiocytic lymphoma
B. Lymphoblastic lymphoma
C. Premyelocytic leukemia
D. CLL

56. **Cavitating lung lesions are seen in following except: Rajasthan 1998**
A. Osteosarcoma B. Histoplasma
C. Silicosis D. Sarcoidosis

57. **Opaque hemithorax is seen in: PGI 1993; 1995**
A. Emphysema thoracis
B. Bronchopneumonia
C. Aspiration of Foreign body
D. Hypoplasia lungs

58. **The Number of bronchopulmonary segments in man is : TN 1998**
A. 12 on Rt side, 11 on Lt side
B. 12 on Rt side, 10 on Lt side
C. 10 of each side
D. 10 on Rt side, 8 on Lt side

59. **Pneumomediastinum can be seen in all except : DNB 1991**
A. Legionnaire's disease B. Ketoacidosis
C. Histiocytosis D. Duodenal perforation
E. Respiratory distress syndrome

60. **The most common type of carcinoma lung in females and non-smokers is: DNB 1990**
A. Squamous cell carcinoma
B. Adenocarcinoma
C. Small cell
D. Large cell

61. **The following diseases generally affect the lower zones except: AP 1986**
A. Asbestosis B. Eosinophilic granuloma
C. Scleroderma D. Rheumatoid arthritis

62. **The following are interstitial disease of large lung volumes except: PGI 1986**
A. Cystic fibrosis
B. Eosinophilic granuloma
C. Lymphangiomyomatosis
D. None of the above

63. **The differential diagnosis of Honey comb lung include the following : AIIMS 1984, 86**
A. Eosinophilic granuloma
B. Sarcoidosis
C. Pneumonconiosis
D. All of the above

64. **Bronchorrhea is characteristically seen in : DNB 1990**
A. Sarcoidosis
B. Scleroderma
C. Bronchoalveolar carcinoma
D. Goodpasture's syndrome

Ans.	48. D	49. C	50. D	51. D	52. B	53. D	54. B	55. A	56. D	57. D
	58. D	59. A	60. B	61. B	62. D	63. D	64. C			

65. **Alveolar proteinosis commonly lead to : Delhi 1987**
A. Honeycomb lung
B. Interstitial disease of large lung volume
C. Diffuse air-space disease
D. All of the above

66. **In adults, the commonest lesion in thoracic inlet is : Delhi 1988**
A. Substernal thyroid B. Teratoma
C. Thymoma D. Lymphoma

67. **Malignant thymoma most commonly spreads to : AIIMS 1985**
A. Brain B. Spine
C. Pleura D. Liver

68. **About -------- % of patients with thymoma have myasthenia gravis and ---------- % of patients with myasthenia gravis have thymomas : AIIMS 1985**
A. 15, 25 B. 25, 15
C. 50, 15 D. 90, 50

69. **"Golden S" Sign is seen in : DNB 1989**
A. Right upper lobe collapse
B. Left upper lobe collapse
C. Right middle lobe collapse
D. Lower lob collapse

70. **Maximal coronal diameters of trachea in males and females are ------ mm respectively : AIIMS 1997**
A. 25, 23 B. 27, 25
C. 25, 21 D. 23, 20

71. **Translucent hemithorax on chest X-ray is seen in: Delhi 1994**
A. Senile emphysema
B. Fallot's tetralogy
C. Pulmonary hypertension
D. Poliomyelitis

72. **Recurrent pneumothoracis is associated with the following except : PGI 1984**
A. Scleroderma B. Histiocytosis
C. Apical pleural bulla D. Endometriosis
E. None of the above

73. **All are superior mediastinal tumors except: PGI 1994**
A. Thymoma
B. Pleurodermoid cyst
C. Branchial cyst
D. Extra-adrenal phaeochromocytoma

74. **Anterior displacement of the trachea may be due to all of the following except: DNB 1990**
A. Mediastinitis
B. Achalasia Cardia
C. Zenker's diverticulum
D. Neuroenteric Cyst
E. Aneurysm of ascending aorta

75. **In pulmonary sarcoidosis, the most prodominant finding in X-ray chest is involvement of : AIIMS 1986**
A. Right paratracheal lymph nodes
B. Lungs in a symmetrical fashion
C. Lungs in asymmetrical fashion
D. Mediastinal Nodes
E. Lung parenchyma and mediastinal nodes

76. **Perihilar fluffy opacities on chest X-ray are seen in: JIPMER 1992**
A. Pulmonary venous hypertension
B. Pulmonary arterial hypertension
C. Pulmonary embolism
D. Pericardial effusion

77. **Best position for chest X-ray to detect left pleural effusion is : Delhi 1986, 87; AIIMS 1992; AI 1993**
A. Right lateral decubitus B. Left lateral decubitus
C. Left lateral D. Supine

78. **In Emphysema, chest X-ray shows : AIIMS 1992**
A. Nodular opacity
B. Increased bronchovascular markings
C. Multiple cystic airways
D. Wide intercostal spaces

79. **Kerley-B-Lines are seen when pulmonary venous pressure is : JIPMER 1993**
A. 8 mm Hg B. 20 mm Hg
C. 25 mm Hg D. 40 mm Hg

80. **The investigation of choice for minimum pericardial effusion is : AI 1993**
A. Lat. decubitus X-ray B. Ultrasound
C. Echocardiography D. ECG

81. **Air bronchogram is seen in: Delhi 1993; PGI 96, 97**
A. Lung abscess B. Lung cavity
C. Pneumothorax D. Consolidation

82. **Middle lobe postural drainage is done in which position: Delhi 1993**
A. Lateral decubitus
B. Supine
C. Prone
D. Sitting and bending forward

83. **'Apical cap sign' is seen in : DNB 1995**
A. Supravalvular AS
B. PDA
C. Mesothelioma
D. Extrapleural haematoma

Ans.	65. C	66. A	67. C	68. C	69. A	70. B	71. D	72. E	73. C	74. E
	75. B	76. A	77. B	78. D	79. C	80. C	81. D	82. A	83. D	

84. Right lung is seen best in the following view: **AIIMS 1984**

A. Right posterior oblique
B. Right anterior oblique
C. Left anterior oblique
D. Lateral

85. Pleural effusion without evident lung infiltration is most often due to : **Delhi 1983**

A. Viral pleurisy B. Carcinoma
C. Lymphoma D. Tuberculosis

86. Tracheal bifurcation is best visualised on which standard view of the chest: **AIIMS 1985**

A. Left anterior oblique B. Left posterior oblique
C. Right anterior oblique D. Right post. oblique

87. Inversion of left hemidiaphragm and paradoxical movement may be due to : **Delhi 1984, 89**

A. Pleural fibrosis
B. Cardiomegaly
C. Diaphragmatic paralysis
D. Pleural fluid

88. X-ray of ant. mediastinum does not show : **UPSC 1985, 86; Delhi 1996, 2001**

A. Teratoma B. Neurofibroma
C. Thymic tumors D. Pleuropericardial cyst

89. Patchy consolidation with hilar lymphadenitis in a child is due to : **NIMHANS 1987**

A. Tuberculosis B. Whooping cough
C. Measles D. All of the above

90. Most common cause for pneumothorax is : **AP 1989**

A. Penetrating trauma
B. Mechanical ventilation
C. Diffuse pulmonary disease
D. Spontaneous

91. Pleural calcification is seen in : **Delhi 1996**

A. Asbestosis B. Bronchiectasis
C. MS D. Pulm. eosinophilia

92. Modified lateral decubitus radiograph of chest can detect pleural fluid in the order of —— ml : **AIIMS 1985**

A. 5-10 B. 10-15
C. 15-25 D. Above 25

93. Severe fat embolism is associated with radiological findings resembling : **AIIMS 1994**

A. Pulmonary Oedema B. Pleural effusion
C. Pulmonary Infarction D. All of the above

94. Right side of mediastinal shadow is formed by all except : **AI 1995**

A. RV
B. Left brachiocephalic vein
C. RA
D. IVC

95. Commonest posterior mediastinal mass is : **AI 1995**

A. Neurogenic tumours
B. Lymphoma
C. Pericardial cysts
D. Aneurysms

96. In chest X-ray, irregular calcification is because of : **PGI 1996**

A. Echinococcal cyst B. Hamartoma
C. Bronchiectasis D. Bronchial adenoma

97. Unilateral elevation of diaphragm is commonly due to: **PGI 1981**

A. Obesity B. Large liver
C. Scoliosis D. Congenital causes

98. Hemoptysis and haematuria, pulmonary infiltrates and nephritis suggests: **AIIMS 1981**

A. Uremic pneumonia
B. Collagen disease
C. Good pasture's syndrome
D. Hypernephroma

99. Diagnostic sign in carcinoma lung in Chest X-ray is : **Delhi 1994**

A. Rib erosion
B. Central destruction within the lesion
C. Flattening of diaphragm
D. Elevation of diaphragm

100. Kerley lines are : **Karnataka 1994, 99**

A. Lines caused by Pulmonary fibrosis in TB
B. Lines caused by increased venous channels
C. Lines to study craniovertebral junction
D. Pulmonary lymphatics dilatation in mitral stenosis

101. In uremic lung, there is : **PGI 1998**

A. Pulmonary edema B. Fibrosis
C. Alveolar injury D. CVC liver

102. Extramedullary hemopoiesis is usually manifested in the chest by: **PGI 1981, 90**

A. Mediastinal mass
B. Posterior paravertebral mass
C. Cardiac enlargement
D. Hillar adenopathy.

103. "Signet ring" and "tramlines" on CT Scan is typically seen in : **DNB 1990**

A. Saccular bronchiectasis
B. Fusiform bronchiectasis
C. Varicose bronchiectasis
D. Cystic bronchiectasis

Ans.										
	84. B	85. D	86. A	87. D	88. B	89. D	90. D	91. A	92. A	93. A
	94. B	95. A	96. B	97. C	98. C	99. A	100. D	101. A	102. B	103. B

104. In Williams-Campbell syndrome, there is : AIIMS 1986

A. Structural defect of bronchi
B. Abnormal mucociliary transport
C. Abnormal secretions
D. 1-antitrypsin deficiency

105. Popcorn calcification in chest X-ray is seen in : Delhi 1985; AI 1997

A. Sarcoidosis
B. Hamartoma
C. Legionella pneumonia
D. Congenital cyst

106. A hematoma of lung following trauma present as : AIIMS 1983

A. A cyst
B. Atelectasis
C. Fleural fluid
D. Pneumonitis

107. Honey-comb lung is seen in which of the following neurocutaneous syndrome : TN 1996

A. von Recklinghausen's
B. Sturge-Weber
C. Tuberous sclerosis
D. Von Hippel-Lindau

108. Early change of pulmonary edema in chest X-ray is: Karnataka 1995

A. Batswing appearance
B. Pleural effusion
C. Kerley's-B-lines
D. Ground glass lung field

109. Commonest cause of chylothorax is : DNB 1992

A. Trauma
B. Filariasis
C. Neoplasm
D. Idiopathic

110. Commonest presentation of chronic coccidio-domycosis is : AIIMS 1987

A. Haemoptysis
B. Hilar lymphadenopathy
C. Patchy infiltrates in lower lobes
D. Asymptomatic

111. In right sided chest X-ray, (PA view), hillum is formed by following except : AIIMS 1997

A. Sup. lobe vein
B. Inf. lobe vein
C. Proximal bronchi
D. Pulmonary artery

112. Chickenpox pneumonia is characterised by: PGI 1980; UPSC 1983

A. Nodular infiltrate
B. Basilar infiltrate
C. Linear fibrotic pattern
D. Pulmonary oedema pattern

113. Both superior and inferior suface of the rib notching is seen in : AIIMS 1984, 85

A. Coarctation of Aorta
B. Superior vena caval obstruction
C. Neurofibromatosis
D. Hyperparathyroidism

114. Spot out wrong statement against interstitial pulmonary oedema : AIIMS 1985

A. Kerley's A lines are present
B. Kerley's B lines are present
C. Perihilar haze
D. Vascular marking becomes clear and prominent

115. Coin shadows in chest can be better visualised in : AIIMS 1985, 86

A. Erect penetrating P.A. view of chest
B. Tomography
C. Supine A.P. View of chest
D. Lateral view of chest

116. Solitary nodule in lung can not be: AI 1988; AMC 1989

A. Tuberculoma
B. Neurofibroma
C. Bronchogenic carcinoma
D. Lymphoma

117. The characteristic X-ray feature of pancoast tumour is : AP 1992

A. Coin shadow
B. Apical consolidation
C. Apical mass lesion with erosion of neck of 1 & 2 ribs
D. Hilar mass

118. Jug handle appearance of chest is seen in: AMU 1985

A. TOF
B. MR
C. Pericardial effusion
D. PAH

119. Following are true about histoplasmosis except : Rajasthan 1996

A. Mediastinal widening
B. Miliary spread to other areas of lung
C. Calcified lesions
D. None of the above

120. "Grape-skin" thin-walled cavities are seen in : AIIMS 1985, 86

A. TB
B. Castleman's disease
C. Williams-Campbell syndrome
D. Coccidiodomycosis

121. "Bulging fissure" patten of pneumonia is seen with: AIIMS 1981; DNB 1989; PGI 1999

A. Streptococci
B. Klebsiella
C. Staph. aureus
D. Varicella

122. Incidence of pulmonary metastasis is maximum with: AIIMS 1981

A. Choriocarcinoma
B. Wilm's tumor
C. Ewing's tumor
D. Seminoma

Ans.									
104. A	105. B	106. A	107. C	108. C	109. C	110. A	111. C	112. B	113. C
114. A	115. B	116. D	117. C	118. D	119. D	120. D	121. B	122. A	

123. Mass within a cavity be seen in all except: PGI 1986

A. Mycetoma
B. Abscess
C. Hydatid cyst
D. Squamous cell carcinoma

124. Which is the commonest form of subphrenic abscess: PGI 1981

A. Raised hemidiaphragm
B. Basal consolidation
C. Pleural effusion
D. Subdiaphragmatic calcification

125. Right sided pleural effusion may be seen in all except: AIIMS 1981

A. CHF
B. Pancreatitis
C. Budd Chiari syndrome
D. Transection of proximal thoracic duct

126. Ground glass appearance is not seen in: AI 2001, 2003

A. Hyaline membrane disease
B. Pneumonia
C. Left-to-right shunt
D. Obstructive TAPVC

127. Multiple pleural densities are more often due to: PGI 1985

A. Thymoma
B. Loculated pleural effusion
C. Mesothelioma
D. Metastasis

128. Commonest malignant tumour of chest wall in children is: AMU 1985

A. Neuroblastoma B. Ewing sarcoma
C. Rhabdomiosarcoma D. Lymphosarcoma

129. Cavitatory lesions in lung are seen in following except: AIIMS 1997

A. Malignant melanoma B. Ca cervix
C. Renal cell carcinoma D. Osteosarcoma

130. In a 2 year child, true about thymus are following except: AIIMS 1999

A. Widening of mediastinum on X-ray
B. Shift of trachea
C. Steriod reduce the size
D. Sharp border with snail like appearance

131. Continuous diaphragm is seen in: Kerala 1999

A. Pneumomediastinum
B. Pneumoperitoneum
C. Pneumopericardium
D. Pleural effusion

132. The following can be features of calcification of benign solitary pulmonary nodule except: Kerala 1999

A. Peripheral B. Popcorn
C. Low density D. Lamellar

133. Investigation of choice for minimal bronchiectasis is: AI 1992

A. Plain X-ray chest B. Bronchography
C. Ultrasound chest D. CT scan chest

134. A 56 years old made pt. was found to have 5 cm cavity in the left apex, the age of which was not known, the next investigation to be done is: AI 2000

A. CT
B. Bronchoscopy with brushings with biopsy
C. Bronchography
D. Percutaneous needle aspiration

135. In chest trauma, immediate X-ray shows opaque shadow. The diagnosis is: JIPMER 2000

A. Haemothorax B. Pulmonary contusion
C. Pneumothorax D. Pericardial effusion

136. Hypertranslucency of lung unilaterally is seen in all except: PGI 2000

A. Pneumothorax
B. Resection of mammary gland
C. Pulm. art. obstruction
D. Pneumonectomy

137. In pulm. embolism, findings in perfusion scan is: PGI 2000

A. Perfusion segmental defect
B. Perfusion defect with normal lung scan & radiography
C. Tenting of diaphragm
D. Normal chest scan

138. All of the following indicate malignancy in chest X-ray except: AIIMS 2000

A. Pleural effusion B. Calcification of lesion
C. Mediastinal widening D. Eccentric cavity

139. Regarding tuberculosis which one is true: AIIMS 2000

A. Cavity indicates active infection.
B. Peripheral rim of ring enhancement of involved lobe suggest active infection.
C. Calcification indicates healed disease.
D. Commonly associated with basal lesion.

Ans.									
123. D	124. A	125. C	126. C	127. C	128. B	129. D	130. D	131. A	132. A
133. B	134. B	135. B	136. C	137. A	138. B	139. D			

140. Unilateral hyperinflation of lung is seen in : AIIMS 2000

A. Collapse
B. Congenital lobar emphysema
C. Bronchiectasis
D. Ca lung

141. All of the following cause miliary shadow on X-ray chest except : Delhi 2001

A. Tuberculosis B. Histoplasmosis
C. Coccidiodomycosis D. Wegner granulomatosis

142. X-ray picture in hyaline membrane disease : Rohtak 2001

A. Soap bubble appearance
B. Honey limb appearance
C. Reticular granulates appearance
D. None

143. More of lower lobe lesions are seen in : Kerala 2001

A. TB B. Silicosis
C. Asbestosis D. CF

144. Bat wing appearance of CXR is due to : DNB 1991; Rohtak 2001

A. Cardiogenic pulmonary edema
B. TB plural effusion
C. Meig's syndrome
D. Bronchogenic carcinoma

145. On X-ray examination of a solitary pulmonary nodule which of the following favours a benign nature : SGPGI 2002

A. Eccentric calcification
B. Bulls eye calcification
C. Lesion is associated with atelectasis
D. Associated with pleural effusion

146. Residual mediastinal/retroperitoneal lymphoma is best assessed by : JIPMER 2002

A. Gallium scan
B. Tech-99m pyrophosphate
C. Restaging procedure
D. Bipedal lymphangiography

147. Air crescent sign on X-ray chest is in : CMC 2001, 2004

A. Lung abscess B. Adenoma lung
C. Aspergilloma D. TB

148. Bedford's sign is : AP 2002

A. Splaying of cranial angle
B. Elevation of left main-stem bronchus
C. Leftward shifting of aorta
D. Seen in left ventricular enlargement

149. A young man with pulmonary tuberculosis presents with massive recurrent hemoptysis. For angiographic treatment, which vascular structure should be evaluated first: AI 2004

A. Pulmonary artery B. Bronchial artery
C. Pulmonary vein D. Superior vena cava

150. A 55 years old man who has been on bed rest for the past 10 days, complains of breathlessness and chest pain. The chest X-ray is normal. The next step in investigation should be: AI 2004

A. Lung Ventilation - perfusion scan
B. Pulmonary arteriography
C. Pulmonary venous wedge angiography
D. Echocardiography

Ans. 140. B 141. D 142. C 143. C 144. A 145. B 146. D 147. C 148. A 149. B 150. A

EXPLANATIONS OF CHEST

1. Ans.— B. Rupture of diaphragm
2. Ans.— C. Benign
3. Ans.— D. Cardiac decompensation
4. Ans.— A. Whipple's disease
5. Ans.— C. Hydatid cyst

   Hydatid cyst (caused by Echinococcus) rarely calcifies in lung.
6. Ans.— D. Goodpasture's syndrome

   Pneumatocele is cystic air collection within lung parenchyma due to obstructive overinflation; occurs during healing process and appears to enlarge while patient improves.
7. Ans.— D. Goodpasture's syndrome
8. Ans.— A. Expiratory films
9. Ans.— D. 25 - 30
10. Ans.— A. Osteosarcoma
11. Ans.— C. Enlarged thyroid
12. Ans.— A. Infarct
13. Ans.— D. Any of the above
14. Ans.— A. Honeycomb lungs

    Staph. pneumothorax, Staph. pneumonia, Trauma, Honey comb lung, Histiocytosis-X, Chemical pneumonitis, Ruptured esophagus.
15. Ans.— A. Children
16. Ans.— D. Cervix
17. Ans.— D. Bronchogenic cyst
18. Ans.— D. Any of the above
19. Ans.— D. There is no growth for at least 2 years.
20. Ans.— A. Squamous
21. Ans.— C. Strength of returning echo
22. Ans.— A. Thickened interlobular septa
23. Ans.— B. Ventilation -perfusion scan

    'Melting sign', Fleishner lines or Hampton Hump may also be seen in Pulmonary embolism with infarction.
24. Ans.— D. Not from the lung`
25. Ans.— C. Lateral decubitus view
26. Ans.— C. Lordotic projection
27. Ans.— A. Aspergillosis
28. Ans.— A. Clear lung fields
29. Ans.— D. Acute pyelonephritis
30. Ans.— D. Full expiration
31. Ans.— B. Markedly well tolerated
32. Ans.— A. Epidermoid carcinoma
33. Ans.— D. Atrial septal defects
34. Ans.— C. Change in calibre of arteries
35. Ans.— B. Displacement of interlobar septum
36. Ans.— C. Intrapulmonary
37. Ans.— B. Lingular segment
38. Ans.— C. Intra-pulmonary pressure is diminished
39. Ans.— B. Infiltrate and nodal enlargement.
40. Ans.— A. Friedlanders pneumonia

    Other pulmonary causes can be infections (fibrotic scars, abscess), vascular (haematoma, AV aneurysms), tumors (Hamartoma, secondaries) and others (broncholits, mitral stenosis). Histoplasmosis causes disseminated small calcified nodules.
41. Ans.— A. Harmartoma
42. Ans.— B. Interstitial air
43. Ans.— C. Cytomegalovirus
44. Ans.— D. Mediastinal shift
45. Ans.— C. Carbon dioxide
46. Ans.— D. Breast
47. Ans.— D. All of the above
48. Ans.— D. Squamous cell carcinoma
49. Ans.— C. Soilicosis
50. Ans.— D. In patient with specific complaints referable to chest.
51. Ans.— D. Rupture of a subpleural bleb
52. Ans.— B. Mitral Stenosis

53. Ans.— D. Squamous cell carcinoma

Other tumors among smokers, may arise in oropharyma, larynx, stomach, liver, bladder etc.

54. Ans.— B. Centriacinar

55. Ans.— A. Diffused histiocytic lymphoma

Anterior Mediastinal masses are mainly 4'T—Thymoma, Teratoma, Thyroid, Terrible Lymphoma (Hodgkin's, NHL).

56. Ans.— D. Sarcoidosis

57. Ans.— D. Hypoplasia lungs

58. Ans.— D. 10 on Rt side, 8 on Lt side

59. Ans.— A. Legionnair's disease

60. Ans.— B. Adenocarcinoma

61. Ans.— B. Eosinophilic granuloma

62. Ans.— D. None of the above

63. Ans.— D. All of the above

64. Ans.— C. Bronchoalveolar carcinoma

65. Ans.— C. Diffuse air-space disease

66. Ans.— A. Substernal thyroid

67. Ans.— C. Pleura

68. Ans.— C. 50, 15

69. Ans.— A. Right upper lobe collapse

70. Ans.— B. 27, 25

71. Ans.— D. Poliomyelitis

72. Ans.— E. None of the above

73. Ans.— C. Branchial cyst

74. Ans.— E. Aneurysm of ascending aorta

75. Ans.— B. Lungs in a symmetrical fashion

76. Ans.— A. Pulmonary venous hypertension

77. Ans.— B. Left lateral decubitus

78. Ans.— D. Wide intercostal spaces

79. Ans.— C. 25 mm Hg

80. Ans.— C. Echocardiography

It is also useful in mitral valve prolapse and aortic stenosis. On Echo, signs of MS are E to F slope of mitral valve decreased (on M mode left atrium dilated, mitral valve orifice narrowed, mitral leaflets thickened; ant. and post. leaflets of mitral valve move parallel and in the same direction.

81. Ans.— D. Consolidation

82. Ans.— A. Lateral decubitus

83. Ans.— D. Extrapleural haematoma

84. Ans.— B. Right anterior oblique

85. Ans.— D. Tuberculosis

86. Ans.— A. Left anterior oblique

87. Ans.— D. Pleural fluid

88. Ans.— B. Neurofibroma

89. Ans.— D. All of the above

90. Ans.— D. Spontaneous

91. Ans.— A. Asbestosis

92. Ans.— A. 5-10

93. Ans.— A. Pulmonary Oedema

94. Ans.— B. Left brachiocephalic vein

Right atrium is best seen on PA or LAO views; Right ventricle on lateral view or right anterior oblique view; left ventricle on lateral view (or Hoffman Rigler sign).

95. Ans.— A. Neurogenic tumours

96. Ans.— B. Hamartoma

97. Ans.— C. Scoliosis

98. Ans.— C. Good pasture's syndrome

99. Ans.— A. Rib erosion

Rib notching of inferior margin is seen in vascular lesions (coarctation, thrombosis, Blalock-Taussig shunt, PS, TOF, Aberrant pulmonary artery, AV fistula, SVC obstruction), neurogenic causes (Inter costal neuroma, neurofibromatosis, Polymyositis, paraplegia) or Osseous lesions (Hyper-parathyroidism (HPH) Thalassemia, Melnick Needles syndrome). Rib notching on superior margin is seen in Rheumatoid arthritis, Scleroderma, SLE, HPH, Restrictive lung disease and Marfan Syndrome.

100. Ans.— D. Pulmonary lymphatics dilatation in mitral stenosis.

101. Ans.— A. Pulmonary edema

102. Ans.— B. Posterior paravertebral mass

103. Ans.— B. Fusiform bronchiectasis

104. Ans.— A. Structural defect of bronchi

105. Ans.— B. Hamartoma

Calcification is seen in 15% and pathognomonic if popcorn type.

106. Ans.— A. A cyst

107. Ans.— C. Tuberous sclerosis

108. Ans.— C. Kerley's B lines

109. Ans.— C. Neoplasm
110. Ans.— A. Haemoptysis
111. Ans.— C. Proximal bronchi
112. Ans.— B. Basilar infiltrate
113. Ans.— C. Neurofibromatosis
114. Ans.— A. Kerley's A lines are present
115. Ans.— B. Tomography
116. Ans.— D. Lymphoma

Other causes include Neoplasm (Pri. lung carcinoma, metastasis, carcinoid), inflammatory (granuloma), vascular (infarct, A-V malformation), congenital bronchogenic cyst, sequestration), miscellaneous (artefact, pseudotumor).

117. Ans.— C. Apical mass lesion with erosion of neck of 1 & 2 ribs.
118. Ans.— D. PAH
119. Ans.— D. None of the above
120. Ans.— D. Coccidiodomycosis
121. Ans.— B. Klebsiella
122. Ans.— A. Choriocarcinoma
123. Ans.— D. Squamous cell carcinoma
124. Ans.— A. Raised hemidiaphragm
125. Ans.— C. Budd Chiari syndrome
126. Ans.— C. Left-to-right shunt
127. Ans.— C. Mesothelioma
128. Ans.— B. Ewing sarcoma
129. Ans.— D. Osteosarcoma
130. Ans.— D. Sharp border with snail like appearance
131. Ans.— A. Pneumomediastinum
132. Ans.— A. Peripheral
133. Ans.— B. Bronchography

Chest films may show linear streaks tram tracks), on-end thickened bronchi, or signet ring deformity, groups of small curvilinear shadows (Grape clusters).

134. Ans.— B. Bronchoscopy with brushings with biopsy

This is to rule out infective, fungal and neoplastic aetiologies.

135. Ans.— B. Pulmonary contusion
136. Ans.— C. Pulm. art. obstruction
137. Ans.— A. Perfusion segmental defect
138. Ans.— B. Calcification of lesion
139. Ans.— D. Commonly associated with basal lesion
140. Ans.— B. Congenital lobar emphysema
141. Ans.— D. Wegner granulomatosis
142. Ans.— C. Reticular granulates appearance
143. Ans.— C. Asbestosis
144. Ans.— A. Cardiogenic pulmonary edema
145. Ans.— B. Bulls eye calcification
146. Ans.— D. Bipedal lymphangiography
147. Ans.— C. Aspergilloma
148. Ans.— A. Splaying of cranial angle
149. Ans.— B. Bronchial artery
150. Ans.— A. Lung Ventilation - perfusion scan

3

IMPORTANT TEXT OF CVS

CARDIOVASCULAR SYSTEM

A. Increased Pulmonary Vascularity

Predominantly Venous

Cor triatriatum sinistrum
Heart failure
Mitral insufficiency
Mitral stenosis
Total anomalous venous return to below diaphragm

Predominantly Arterial

Atrial septal defect
Congenital coronary fistula
Endocardial cushion defects
High output heart
Lutembacher's syndrome
Partial anomalous venous return
Patent ductus arteriosus
Pickwickian obesity
Primary polycythemia
Single ventricle
Taussig-Bing complex
Transposition of great vessels
Truncus arteriosus
Ventricular septal defect

B. Pulmonary Hypertension and Cor Pulmonale

Chronic Hypoxia

Chest deformities
Chronic airway obstruction (adenoids)
High altitude dwelling
Pickwickian obesity

Diffuse Interstitial Lung Disease

Chronic bronchitis
Dermatomyositis
Emphysema
Hamman-Rich syndrome
Idiopathic fibrosis
Lupus erythematosus
Lymphangitic metastases
Mucoviscidosis
Periarteritis nodosa
Pneumoconiosis
Scleroderma
Tuberculosis with extensive fibrosis

Diffuse Pulmonary Arteritis

Idiopathic
Left-to-right shunts (Eisenmenger's physiology)
Mitral stenosis (long standing)
Schistosomiasis

Thromboembolism

Recurrent pulmonary emboli
Sickle cell anemia (pulmonary thrombi)
Hypervolemia of Right Heart
Ventriculoartrial shunt for hydrocephalus

C. High Output Heart

Arteriovenous fistula (extrapulmonary)
Beriberi
Hypervolemia (transfusions, fluid overload)
Paget's disease
Pickwickian obesity
Pregnancy
Primary polycythemia
Pyrexia
Severe anemia
Sickle cell anemia
Thyrotoxicosis

D. Pericardial Effusion

Amoebic pericarditis
Congestive failure
Coxsackie pericarditis
Dissecting aneurysm with leakage
Histoplasmosis
Idiopathic
Lupus erythematosus
Mycotic infection
Myxedema
Neoplastic Pericarditis
Nephrosis
Periarteritis nodosa
Post-coronary artery bypass surgery
Post-myocardial infarction syndrome
Pyogenic infection
Rheumatic fever
Scleroderma
Syphilis
Toxoplasmosis
Trauma
Tuberculosis
Uremia
Viral infections

E. Enlarged Left Atrium

Congenital coronary fistula
Heart failure
Mitral insufficiency
Myocardiopathies
Myxoma of left atrium
Patent ductus arteriosus
Ventricular septal defect

F. Prominent or Enlarged Ascending Aorta and/or Aortic Arch

Aneurysm
Ankylosing spondylitis
Aortic insufficiency
Aortic stenosis
Atherosclerosis
Coarctation of Aorta
Homocystinuria
Marfan's disease
Patent ductus arteriosus
Pseudocoarctation
Pseudoxanthoma elasticum
Syphilitic aortitis
Takayasu's arteritis
Tetralogy of Fallot
Tricuspid atresia without transposition
Truncus arteriosus (type-IV)

G. Cardiac Calcifications

Aneurysm of coronary artery
Aneurysm of sinus of Valsalva
Atrial clot
Coronary atherosclerosis
Left atrium (mitral disease)
Myocardial infarct
Myxoma of atrium
Pericardium
Valvular
Aortic (aortic stenosis)
Mitral annulus

H. Vascular Calcifications

Arterial

Artherosclerosis
Homocystinuria
Hyperparathyroidism
Premature arteriosclerosis
Familial hyperlipemias
Progeria
Secondary hyperlipemia
Cushing's syndrome
Diabetes
Glycogen storage disease
Hypothyroidism
Lipodystrophy
Nephrotic syndrome
Renal homotransplantation
Pseudoxanthoma elasticum
Werner's syndrome

Venous

Arteriovenous malformation
Hemangioma
Maffucci's syndrome
Phleboliths

MCQ's OF CVS

What is important in CVS

Heart (Enlargement of different chambers, Pericardial calcification and effusion, Infarction), Anomalous vasculature

1. **Pericardial calcification is caused by following except : PGI 1982, 86, 99**
   A. Radiotherapy to the mediastinum
   B. Methysergide therapy
   C. Anticoagulant therapy
   D. Benign pericarditis
   E. Dermatomyositis
2. **Hilar dance on fluoroscopy is seen in : PGI 1982; DNB 1990**
   A. ASD B. TOF
   C. VSD D. TGV
3. **On PA view of X-ray chest, cardiac silhoutte is increased in following except : AIIMS 1997**
   A. TOF B. Pericardial effusion
   C. Pleural effusion D. None of the above
4. **Lateral artrial hypertrophy can be detected by barium X-ray in : TN 1996, 98**
   A. A.P. view B. Lateral view
   C. RAO view D. LAO view
5. **In coarctation of Aorta the rib changes are seen from: Karnataka 1995**
   A. 1-12th B. 3-6th
   C. 4-9th D. 8-12th
6. **Calcification of ascending aorta is commonly caused by all except : AMU 1986, 91**
   A. Atherosclerosis B. Syphilis
   C. Hypertension D. Hypercholesterolemia
7. **"Tulip bulb aorta" is typically seen in —— syndrome: AIIMS 1985, 89**
   A. Down's B. Marfan's
   C. Eisenmenger's D. Turner's
8. **Flask shaped heart is seen in the following except : PGI 1997**
   A. Ebstein's anomaly B. TOF
   C. Pericardial effusion D. None
9. **Which of the following is pathognomonic of Pulmonary arterial hypertension : AIIMS 1986**
   A. Dilatation of pulmonary trunk
   B. Calcification of central Pulm. vessels
   C. Normal sized heart
   D. Rapid tapering of Pulmonary arteries
10. **Cottage leaf appearance is seen in : AIIMS 1982**
    A. TOF B. TAPVD
    C. TAPAD D. MS
11. **Egg in cup appearance is seen in : DNB 1989**
    A. TOF
    B. MR
    C. Constrictive pericarditis
    D. Transposition of great vessels
12. **In long standing mitral stenosis, the pulmonary vessels are : AIIMS 1983**
    A. Diminished in lower lung
    B. Diminished in upper lung
    C. Diminished in midlung
    D. Enlarged in lower lung
13. **False about myocardial perfusion scan is : Rajasthan 1996**
    A. Localization of site of infarction
    B. Detection of infarction
    C. Differentiates between old & recent infarcts
    D. None of the above
14. **Stag Antlers sign is seen in : AIIMS 1994**
    A. PAH B. PVH
    C. TOF D. Pulm. oedema
15. **Non-viable part of myocardium is diagnosed by following except : UP 1998**
    A. Tc99 scintigraphy
    B. Thallium scintigraphy
    C. Positron emission tomography
    D. Standard CT
16. **Following signs are seen in pericardial effusion except : AIIMS 1983, 86, 90**
    A. Water bottle configuration
    B. Fat pad sign
    C. Stag Antler sign
    D. Differential density sign

Ans.	1. E	2. A	3. A	4. B	5. B	6. C	7. B	8. B	9. B	10. C
	11. C	12. A	13. C	14. B	15. D	16. C				

17. **Most common radiation induced heart disease following high dose radiotherapy to the thorax is : AMC 1983, 89, 92**
A. Pericarditis B. Cardiac atrophy
C. Intracardiac thrombi D. None of the above

18. **Characteristic radiographic finding in ASD is : AIIMS 1993**
A. Enlarged left atrium
B. Pulmonary plethora
C. Pulmonary artery hypertension
D. Enlarged left ventricle

19. **Commonest site of calcification in constrictive pericarditis is : AI 1995**
A. Left border LA B. AV groove
C. Right border RA D. Right ventricle

20. **Cardiac activity of the fetus seen in Ultrasound by : TN 1999**
A. 4 weeks B. 5 weeks
C. 6 weeks D. 7 weeks

21. **Left-to-right shunt is usually demonstrated in chest X-rays by : PGI 1982; AIIMS 1984**
A. Increase in pulmonary venous markings
B. Increase in size of pulmonary arteries
C. Increase in number of pulmonary arteries
D. Increase in pulmonary vascular markings

22. **Superior vena cava syndrome is treated by : WB 1998**
A. External beam radiation
B. Steroid
C. Intra-cavitatory/brachy therapy
D. All

23. **First investigation of choice of diagnosis of pericardial effusion is : AI 1988; DNB 1990**
A. Angiocardiography
B. Echocardiography
C. Compound tomography
D. Magnetic resonance imaging

24. **An aneurysm of the sinus of Valsalva usually arises from : AMU 1988**
A. Right aortic sinus
B. Left aortic sinus
C. Posterior aortic sinus
D. Pulmonary outflow tract
E. Right Ventricle

25. **One can easily distinguish Right atrium from Right ventricular enlargement on X-ray in : AP 1989**
A. Eisenmenger's complex
B. Tricuspid stenosis
C. Ebstein disease
D. All of the above

26. **Pericardial cysts are more common in : TN 1989**
A. Right apex
B. Left apex
C. Right cardiophrenic angle
D. Left cardiophrenic angle

27. **During angiocardiography the mitral valve is best visualized in : NIMHANS 1986**
A. Lateral view
B. Frontal view
C. Right anterior oblique view
D. None of the above

28. **Fluoroscopy may be used in the diagnosis of all of the following except : JIPMER 1998**
A. Coronary artery calcification
B. Diaphragmatic palsy
C. Valve calcification
D. LV function

29. **The overall heart size in tetralogy of Fallot is usually: AMU 1989**
A. Markedly enlarged
B. Normal or relatively small
C. Slightly enlarged
D. Moderately enlarged

30. **Cardiac catheterisation was first attempted by : AIIMS 1983, 87**
A. Phillip Bozzini B. Gustav Killian
C. Dulius Bruck D. Warner Forssman

31. **Roentgenographic microcardia is not a characteristic of : AIIMS 1983**
A. Addison's disease
B. Malnutrition
C. Endocardial fibroelastosis
D. None of the above

32. **Complete heart-block is demonstrated radiologically as : PGI 1981**
A. Pulmonary vascular engorgement sometimes
B. Right ventricular and left atrial enlargement
C. Mostly left ventricular enlargement, cardiomegaly
D. All of the above

33. **Radiologic findings of paroxysmal tachycardia are : AIIMS 1982**
A. Pulmonary congestion
B. Rapid and feeble cardiac pulsation
C. Non-specific cardiomegaly of varying degree
D. All are true

34. **In frontal view of an oesophagram of an infant there is usually no aortic impression. A marked impression suggests : AIIMS 1981**
A. Aortic stenosis
B. Truncus arteriosus
C. Persistent ductus arteriosus
D. All of the above

Ans.									
17. A	18. B	19. D	20. D	21. D	22. A	23. B	24. A	25. C	26. C
27. C	28. A	29. B	30. D	31. C	32. D	33. D	34. D		

3.6 RADIOLOGY

35. **Calcification in the heart wall is suggestive of : JIPMER 1992**
A. Dressler's syndrome
B. Scleroderma
C. Fibroelastosis
D. Endomyocardial fibrosis

36. **Following are radiological changes in Tetralogy of Fallot except : JIPMER 1993**
A. Prominent cardiac apex
B. Cardiomegaly
C. Prominent pulmonary trunk
D. Normal right atrial shadow

37. **Isotopes used in myocardial perfusion scan is : TN 1993, 97**
A. Technitium
B. Thallium
C. Stannous pyrophosphate
D. Gallium

38. **Right retrocardiac space is best seen on which view : AIIMS 1985**
A. Lateral
B. Left anterior oblique
C. Right posterior oblique
D. Right anterior oblique

39. **In mitral stenosis, the presence of left atrial wall calcification implies : AIIMS 1982**
A. No correlation at all
B. A low incidence of left atrial thrombosis
C. A high incidence of left atrial thrombosis
D. Incidence of right atrial thrombosis

40. **'Silent Heart' on fluoroscopy is seen in the following except : AIIMS 1985**
A. Mitral incompetence B. Periacardial effusion
C. Ebstein anomaly D. Cardiomyopathy

41. **Aortic dissection is best diagnosis by : AI 1996**
A. CT Scan B. Angiography
C. Chest X-ray D. Digital substraction

42. **Match List-I correctly with List-II and select the correct answer using the codes given below the lists : TNPSC 1998**

List-I	List-II
A. Right ventricle	1. RAO view
B. Right atrium	2. Lat. view
C. Left atrium	3. PA view & LAO view
D. Left ventricle	4. PA view

Codes :

	a	b	c	d
A.	1	2	3	4
B.	2	3	1	4
C.	3	4	2	1
D.	4	1	3	2

43. **All the following are radiological features of mitral stenosis except : AIIMS 2000**
A. Straight left heart border
B. Oligemia of upper lung fields
C. Pulmonary hemosiderosis
D. Lifting of the left bronchus

44. **Following are seen in CCF exept : AI 2000**
A. Kerley B lines
B. Enlarged pulmonary artery markings
C. Enlarged lower lobe veins
D. Pleural effusion

45. **Enlarged left atrium on X-ray shows all except : AIIMS 2002**
A. Double shadow.
B. Right lateral view shows obliteration of retrosternal shadow.
C. Lifting of left bronchus.
D. Posterior displacement of oesophagus on barium swallow.

46. **Boot shaped heart with oligemia is seen in : SGPGI 2002**
A. TGA B. TOF
C. ASD D. PDA

47. **Radiological signs of co-arctation of aorta without cardiac failure are all except : UP 2002**
A. Rib notching B. 'E 'sign
C. Normal shaped heart D. Egg on side appearance

48. **T_1 and T_2 images are a feature of which diagnostic test: Karnataka 2004**
A Ultrasound B C.T. scan
C Duplex scan D MRI scan

49. **In which of the following a 'Cour-en-Sabot' shape of the heart is seen : AI 2004**
A. Tricuspid atresia
B. Ventricular septal defect
C. Transposition of great arteries
D. Tetralogy of Fallot

50. **Potential for Reperfusion of the tissue, post-infarct can be assessed by : AI 2009**
A. MUGA scan B. Thallium scan
C. Echo cardiography D. MRI

Ans. 35. A 36. B 37. B 38. D 39. C 40. B 41. D 42. B 43. B 44. C 45. D 46. B 47. D 48. D 49. D 50. B

EXPLANATIONS OF CVS

1. Ans.— E. Dermatomyositis
2. Ans.— A. ASD
3. Ans.— A. TOF
4. Ans.— B. Lateral view
5. Ans.— B. 3-6th
6. Ans.— C. Hypertension
7. Ans.— B. Marfan's
8. Ans.— B. TOF
9. Ans.— B. Calcification of central Pulm. vessels
10. Ans.— C. TAPAD
11. Ans.— C. Constrictive pericarditis
12. Ans.— A. Diminished in lower lung
13. Ans.— C. Differentiates between old & recent infarcts
14. Ans.— B. PVH
15. Ans.— D. Standard CT

    9c labelled RBC's are used and quantification and volume of each ventricle is measured.
16. Ans.— C. Stag Antler sign
17. Ans.— A. Pericarditis
18. Ans.— B. Pulmonary plethora
19. Ans.— D. Right ventricle

    Right heart is mainly involved leading to the clinical features of right heart failure. Pericardial calcification is best seen on lateral view, is present in 50% cases.
20. Ans.— D. 7 weeks
21. Ans.— D. Increase in pulmonary vascular markings
22. Ans.— A. External beam radiation
23. Ans.— B. Echocardiography

    Echocardiography can differentiate pericardial effusion from cardiomyopathy, myxoma and other cardiac abnormalities. Signs on Echocardiography includes separation of epicardial and pericardial echoes; flattening of normal pericardial motion; temponade (exaggerated ant. RV wall motion) and pericardial fat appears hypoechoic.
24. Ans.— A. Right aortic sinus
25. Ans.— C. Ebstein disease
26. Ans.— C. Right cardiophrenic angle
27. Ans.— C. Right anterior oblique view

    It is also useful in mitral valve prolapse and aortic stenosis. On Echo, signs of MS are E to F slope of mitral valve decreased (on M mode left atrium dilated, mitral valve orifice narrowed, mitral leaflets thickened; ant. and post. leaflets of mitral valve move parallel and in the same direction).
28. Ans.— A. Coronary artery calcification
29. Ans.— B. Normal or relatively small
30. Ans.— D. Warner Forssman
31. Ans.— C. Endocardial fibroelastosis
32. Ans.— D. All of the above
33. Ans.— D. All are true
34. Ans.— D. All of the above
35. Ans.— A. Dressler's syndrome

    Dressler's syndrome (less than 4% incidence) also called Post MI syndrome, aetiology is autoimmune reaction, onset in 2-3 weeks (range 1 week to several months) following MI, relapses occur as late as 2 years after initial episode, fever, pericarditis (+ pericardial effusion), pleuritis (+ pleural effusion) and pneumonitis.
36. Ans.— B. Cardiomegaly
37. Ans.— B. Thallium
38. Ans.— D. Right anterior oblique
39. Ans.— C. A high incidence of left atrial thrombosis

40. Ans.— B. Periacardial effusion

41. Ans.— D. Digital substraction

It is of first choice. In angiography, there are double barrel aorta sign (in 87%) linear translucency, compression of true lumen, AR, distorted aortic wall.

42. Ans.— B. 2 3 1 4

43. Ans.— B. Oligemia of upper lung fields

44. Ans.— C. Enlarged lower lobe veins

Enlarged particular chambers characteristic of lesion responsible for failure, redistribution to apices and elevated pulmonary vascular pressures, pleural effusions with associated interlobar effusions may be seen.

45. Ans.— D. Posterior displacement of oesophagus on barium swallow

46. Ans.— B. TOF

47. Ans.— D. Egg on side appearance

48. Ans.— D. MRI scan

49. Ans.— D. Tetralogy of Fallot

50. Ans. B. Thallium scan

* Measurement of increased pulmonary uptake.
* Less hepatobiliary and bowel uptake.
* Detection of resting ischemia (hibernating myocardium/reversible myocardial damage).
* Thallium scan produces cold spot in MI i.e. it is taken by healthy tissue. So, it detects old infarcted area.
* Produces pyrophosphate scan produces hot spot is acute MI i.e. it detects fresh infarcted area.

4

IMPORTANT TEXT OF GIT

PNEUMATOSIS INTESTINALIS

= multiple thin=walled, non-communicating, gas filled cysts located in subserosa = submucosa with a normal mucosa + muscularis

1. Primary Pneumatosis Intestinalis (15%)
2. Secondary Pneumatosis Intestinalis (85%)

Causes:

A. *Ischemia*
   1. Necrotizing enterocolitis
   2. Mesenteric vascular disease

B. *Trauma*
   1. Ingestion of corrosives
   2. Gastrointestinal endoscopy
   3. Jejunoileal bypass surgery

C. *Infection*
   1. Primary infection of bowel wall
   2. Intestinal parasites
   3. Perforated jejunal diverticulum

D. *Inflammation*
   1. Pyloric/duodenal ulcer
   2. Inflammatory bowel disease
   3. Connective tissue disease
   4. Whipple disease

E. *Pulmonary causes*
   1. Emphysema
   2. Bullous disease of lung
   3. Chronic bronchitis
   4. Asthma

F. *Colonic Obstruction*

* Asymptomatic
* Radiolucent clusters of cysts along contour of bowel wall.
* Polypoid defects in barium column = pneumoperitoneum

SOAP BUBBLE APPEARANCE IN ABDOMEN OF NEONATE

1. Feces in infant fed by mouth
2. Meconium ileus
3. Meconium plug : Gas in and around plug, in distribution of colon
4. Necrotizing enterocolitis : submucosal pneumatosis
5. Atresia/severe stenosis: pneumatosis
6. Hirschsprung disease

ACHALASIA PATTERN

= Megasophagus

1. Idiopathic achalasia
2. Changes disease : Patients commonly from South America; often associated with megacolon + cardiomegaly.
3. Infiltrating lesion of distal esophagus/gastric cardia (e.g., carcinoma).
4. Amyloidosis : Associated with macroglossia, thickened small bowel folds.
5. Idiopathic intestinal pesudo obstruction = degeneration of innervation.
6. Presbyesophagus
7. Ehlers-Danlos syndrome
8. Postvagotomy syndrome
9. Scleroderma

AIR ESOPHAGRAM

1. Normal vari ant
2. Scleroderma
3. Distal obstruction tumor, stricture, achalasia
4. Thoracic surgery
5. Mediastinal inflammatory disease
6. S/P total laryngectomy (esophageal speech)
7. Endotracheal intubation + PEEP

DOUBLE-BARREL ESOPHAGUS

1. Dissecting intramural hematoma from emetogenic injury.
2. Mallory-Weiss tear trauma, esophagoscopy (in 0.25%), bougiage (in 0.5%), ingestion of foreign bodies, spontaneous (bleeding diathesis).
3. Intramural bascess
4. Intraluminal diverticulum
5. Esophageal duplication (in communication with esophageal lumen present).

BULL'S EYE LESIONS

A. Primary Neoplasms
   1. Leiomyoma, leiomyosarcoma
   2. Lymphoma
   3. Carcinoid
   4. Primary carcinoma

B. Hematogenous Metastasis
   1. Malignant melanoma : Usually spares large bowel
   2. Breast cancer (15%) : Scirrhous appearance in stomach
   3. Cancer in lung
   4. Renal cell carcinoma
   5. Kaposi sarcoma
   6. Bladder carcinoma

C. Ectopic pancreas to duodenum/stomach

D. Eosinophilic Granuloma most frequently in stomach

COLONIC THUMBPRINTING

= Sharply defined fingerlike marginal indentations at contours of wall.

1. Ischemia + Ischemic colitis
   Occulusive vascular disease, hypercoagulability state, hemorrhage into bowel wall (bleeding diathesis, anticoagulants,) traumatic intramural hematoma.
2. Inflammation : Ulcerative colitis, Crohn colitis
3. Infection : Acute amebiasis, schistosomiasis, strongyloidiasis, cytomegalovirus (in renal transplant recipients), pseudomembranous colitis.
4. Malignant Lesions : Localized primary lymphoma, hematogenous metastasis.
5. Miscellaneous : Endometriosis, amyloidosis, pneumatosis intestinalis, diverticulosis, diverticulitis, herediatary angioneurotic.

DDX BETWEEN CROHN DISEASE VERSUS ULCERATIVE COLITIS

mnemonic: "LUCIFERM

	Crohn's Disease	*Ulcerative Colitis*
Location	right side	left side
Ulcers	deep	shallow
Contraction	no	yes
Ileocecal valve	thickened	gaping
Fistulae	yes	no
Eccentricity	yes	no
Rate of carcinoma	slight increase	marked increase
Megacolon	unusual	yes

MCQ's OF GIT

What is important in GIT

Oesophagus (Achalasia, Carcinoma), Stomach and Duodenum (Ulcer, Carcinoma, Duodenal atresia, Carcinoma), Jejunum, Ileum (Atresia), Large bowel (Diverticulosis, Carcinoma, Megacolon), Intestinal obstruction, Crohn's, Ulcerative colitis, T.B., Amoebiasis, Liver (Enlargement, Masses), Gall bladder (Stones, Calcification), Pancreas (Tumours), Spleen (Rupture, Masses)

1. In a patient with infiltration of spleen by lymphoma or leukaemia, the spleen scan shows : AIIMS 1982, 85, 93

A. Normal splenic sequestration
B. Increased splenic sequestration
C. Decreased splenic sequestration
D. None of the above

2. The most important radiological features of chronic gastric ulcer is all except : ESI 1986

A. Gastrospasm
B. Localised tenderness of pressure
C. Demonstration of ulcer crate
D. Central fleck of barium with periphery devoid of barium
E. Convergence of mucosal ruga

3. "Ulcer Crater" on barium X-ray examination indicates the diagnosis of : AIIMS 1991, 96

A. Gastric Carcinoma
B. Duodenal ulcer
C. Duodenal diverticulum
D. Duodenal stricture

4. Aneurysm of abdominal aorta is diagnosed by : AIIMS 1986; AI 1987, 92

A. Ultrasonography
B. Clinical examination
C. Lateral X-ray of the abdomen
D. History

5. Feathery appearance in jejunum is due to : PGI 1999

A. Valvulæ conniventes B. Haustrations
C. Luminal gas D. Vascular network

6. "Football sign" is seen in : AIIMS 1985

A. Porcelain GB B. Ascites
C. Pneumoperitoneum D. Portal vein thrombosis

7. When an individual is frightened or emotionally disturbed, the stomach tends to be : AIIMS 1982

A. Not effected B. Contracts irregularly
C. Hypertonic D. Hypotonic

8. Dilated jejunal loops on plain X-ray Abdomen are identified by : JIPMER 1992

A. Haustrations B. Valvulae conniventes
C. Characterless bowel D. Air fluid levels

9. The contrast used in liver scan is : JIPMER 1992

A. I131 Rose Bengal B. Biligraffin
C. Technetium 99 D. Gallium 238

10. X-ray findings characteristic of small intestinal malabsorption syndrome are all of the following except : JIPMER 1992

A. Flocculation of barium B. Dilatation of bowel
C. Increased transit time D. Mucosal atrophy

11. X-ray findings suggestive of Achalasia cardia are following except : JIPMER 1992, 93

A. Megaesophagus
B. Tortuous esophagus
C. Fluid level in esophagus
D. Diverticulum in esophagus

12. Minimal ascities can be detected by : AIIMS 1992

A. X-ray B. USG
C. CT scan D. MRI

13. Following are associated with gas within colonic wall except : JIPMER 1993

A. Pneumatosis coli
B. Necrotizing enterocolitis
C. Hirschsprungs disease
D. COPD

14. Abdominal organ best suited for CT scanning : AIIMS 1985, 90; TN 1996, 98

A. Liver B. Gall bladder
C. Pancreas D. Kidneys

15. Technetium labelled RBC's are used for : AI 1995

A. Radioimaging of biliary tree
B. Pulm. embolism
C. Renal disease
D. Splenic disease

Ans.									
1. C	2. C	3. B	4. A	5. A	6. C	7. D	8. B	9. C	10. C
11. D	12. C	13. C	14. C	15. D					

16. Which of the following is the least useful investigation in haematemesis : PGI 1983; AIIMS 1986

A. Barium meal
B. Selective arteriography
C. Radioactive nucleotide scanning
D. Endoscopy

17. In radiology, small intestine obstruction is identified by : PGI 1983

A. Valvae conniventes B. Haustrations
C. Peripheral location D. None of the above

18. Which is the commonest sign of subphrenic abscess : PGI 1984

A. Raised hemidiaphragm
B. Basal consolidation
C. Pleural effusion
D. Subdiaphragmatic calcification

19. Phrygian cap is feature of the : AMU 1986, 91

A. Pancreas B. Gall bladder
C. Kidney D. Stomach

20. Poor visualisation of gall bladder has been noted in : AIIMS 1985

A. Fat free diet
B. Non-tropical sprue
C. Metachromatic leukogystrophy
D. Chronic idiopathic jaundice
E. All are true

21. Sub-diaphragmatic abscess may show all except : AIIMS 1980; AMC 1987

A. Diaphragm is fixed
B. Diaphragm is pulled-up
C. Blunted costophrenic angle
D. Pleural effusion may occur
E. Sub-phrenic gas shadow is diagnostic

22. 'Sentinel loop' on X-ray is seen in : AP 1997

A. Acute pancreatitis B. Pancreatic mass
C. Splenomegaly D. Carcinoma colon

23. X-ray finding in metastatic carcinoma to mesentery and gut are all except : AIIMS 1983

A. Folds are angulated in their tips.
B. Thinning of bowel wall.
C. There will be oedema.
D. Immediate adjoining valvulae may appear spiked.
E. If metastasis invades, the mucosa ulceration produced.

24. X-ray features of lymphoma of stomach are all except : AIIMS 1981

A. Broad ulceration
B. Moderate rigidity
C. Peristalsis remain undisturbed
D. Fingerprint impression pattern due to diffuse intramural invasion

25. "Inverted-V sign is seen in outlining of : AIIMS 1985

A. Medial umbilical ligament
B. One lateral umbilical ligament
C. Both lateral umbilical ligament
D. Intestinal perforation

26. Contrast media of choice in investigating a suspected case of ileal perforation : AIIMS 1983

A. Barium sulphate B. Gastrograffin
C. Dionosil viscous D. Lipoidol

27. "Mustache sign" is typically present in : DNB 1991

A. Splenosis
B. Gas under hemidiaphragm
C. Achalasia cardia
D. Ascites

28. Barium meal picture in a pseudocyst of the pancreas shows : Karnataka 1989

A. Filling defect in the stomach
B. A ball like radio opaque shadow in the abdomen
C. Stomach displaced forwards
D. Contracted stomach

29. Gas under diaphragm is seen in X-ray abdomen in all of the following ruptures except : AI 1990; PGI 1993

A. Appendicular B. Duodenal ulcer
C. Intestinal D. Subphrenic abscess

30. 'Scalloping' of the edge of sigmoid colon on barium enema is seen in : AP 1997

A. Diverticulosis
B. Ulcerative colitis
C. Carcinoma colon
D. Pneumatosis intestinalis

Match the following (31-33) : AIIMS 1982

A. Carman's sign B. Ulcus callosum
C. Handek's niche

31. Classical ulcer crater as outlined by barium inprofile :

32. A chronic ulcer producing induration of gastric wall :

33. A menisocoid shaped ulcer crater produced by an intralumin gastric tumour surrounding it and separating it from barium filled stomach :

34. In hypertrophic pyloric stenosis, most useful is : Delhi 2000

A. Ba follow through B. USG
C. Ba meal D. CT Scan

35. Widening of the C-loop in X-ray is diagnostic of : AIIMS 1982

A. Chronic pancreatitis
B. Carcinoma head of pancreas
C. Periampullary carcinoma
D. Calculi in the ampulla of Vater

Ans.										
	16. B	17. A	18. A	19. A	20. E	21. C	22. A	23. B	24. C	25. C
	26. B	27. B	28. C	29. D	30. D	31. C	32. B	33. A	34. B	35. B

36. Most sensitive investigation of pancreatic carcinoma is : PGI 1983

A. Angiography B. ERCP
C. Ultrasound D. CT Scan

37. Best investigation for small bowel tumor is : JIPMER 1998

A. Enteroclysis
B. Barium meal follow through
C. Ultrasound
D. CT

38. Inverted 'U' shaped grossly dilated gasfilled loop of colon in straight X-ray abdomen is seen in : BHU 1985; DNB 1998

A. Volvulus of colon
B. Intussusception
C. Fulminant ulcerative colitis
D. All of the above

39. Splenic calcification occurs in : BHU 1985

A. Coeliac disease B. Gaucher disease
C. Brucellosis D. Malaria

40. In an infant who is clinically obstructed, the radiologist reports 'double bubble sign'. The most likely diagnosis is : AIIMS 1986

A. Duodenal atresia
B. Annular pancreas
C. Formation on band across the duodenum
D. All of the above

41. Coiled spring appearance on barium enema is seen in : PGI 1995; Delhi 1998

A. Carcinoma colon B. Sigmoid volvulus
C. Intussusception D. Ileal atresia

42. The most common cause of neonatal haemoperitoneum is : AMU 1987

A. Rupture of hydronephrotic calyx
B. Necrotising enterocolitis
C. Trauma
D. Exchange transfusion via umbilical catheter
E. Haemorrhagic disease of newborn

43. Rectal atresia is often associated with : PGI 1986

A. Rectovaginal communication
B. Rectovesical communication
C. A patent anus
D. Duodenal obstruction
E. Failure of proper descent of the hindgut

44. Severe chest pain with hematemesis and dysphagia, in association with mediastinal emphysema is : PGI 1986

A. Boerhave syndrome
B. Mallory Weiss syndrome
C. Ruptured oesophageal varices
D. Intraumural oesophageal rupture
E. Carcinoma oesophagus

45. The radiological diagnostic features of acute pancreatitis include the following except : AMU 1988; Rajasthan 1996

A. Reverse figure 3 sing
B. Massive left pleural effusion
C. Blurring of left psoas and renal shadows
D. Local or generalized a dynamic ileus
E. On CT scan swelling confined to pancreatic head

46. The method of choice in preliminary evaluation of biliary obstruction with clinical jaundice is : AIIMS 1989

A. Oral cholecystography (OCG)
B. Endoscopic retrograde cholangiopancreatography (ERCP)
C. CT Scan
D. Ultrasonography
E. Intravenous choledochography (IVC)

47. Residue of barium meal is seen in the stomach after 6 hours. This could be due to : DNB 1989

A. Pyloric stenosis B. Hypotonia
C. Pylerospasm D. Any of the above

48. Most specific investigation of acute interstitial pancreatitis is : AIIMS 1985; TN 1996, 98; Orissa 1998; Delhi 2000

A. CT B. ERCP
C. PCT D. USG

49. Following are causes of pseudopneumo peritoneum except : DNB 1998

A. Chiladiti syndrome
B. Uneven diaphragm
C. Peritoneal dialysis
D. Intramural gas in pneumatosis intestinalis

50. Following are causes of gas in the biliary tree except : DNB 1998

A. Gall stone fistula
B. Laxed sphincter
C. Emphysematous cholecystitis
D. Periampullary carcinoma of pancreas

51. Radiological finding in ileal atresia : PGI 2000

A. Microcolon on Ba enema
B. Double-bubble sign
C. Coil spring appearance in Ba enema
D. Obstruction in Ba meal

52. Watermelon stomach results due to : AIIMS 1998

A. Carcinoma B. Leiomyosarcoma
C. Duodenal atresia D. Vascular ectasia

Ans. 36. D 37. A 38. A 39. C 40. D 41. C 42. C 43. C 44. A 45. E
46. D 47. D 48. A 49. C 50. D 51. C 52. D

53. **Barium meal is indicated in : Rajasthan 1994**
A. Gasric outlet obstruction
B. Obstruction of jejunum
C. Obstruction of ileum
D. Obstruction of colon

54. **The following are associated with focal absent activity on splenic scintigraphy except : DNB 1991**
A. Septic emboli B. Cyanotic heart disease
C. Trauma D. Sarcoidosis
E. Thalassaemia

55. **After birth, time taken for air to reach various parts of GIT is : DNB 1997**

	Stomach (hrs)	Caecum	Sigmoid (hrs)	Rectum colon (hrs)
A.	Within sec.	2-3	5-6	Upto 8
B.	Within min.	3-4	8-9	Upto 10
C.	Within min.	3-4	8-9	Upto 12
D.	30-60 min	4-6	8-9	Upto 24

56. **Ileum in barium meal looks like : AIIMS 1984; AMC 1984, 89**
A. Characteristic B. Irregular dilatation
C. Characterless D. None of the above

57. **Thumb-printing appearance on Barium meal is seen in : AIIMS 1982, 85; ESI 1989**
A. Diverticulitis B. Ischemic colitis
C. Ulcerative colitis D. Carcinoma colon

58. **Oral cholecystography is associated with following except : AI 1997**
A. Hepatic function B. More function of GB
C. Water absorption D. Bile composition

59. **Presence of opaque gall stones in children or young adults is usually associated with : AIIMS 1984**
A. Lactate deficiency
B. Hemolytic anemias
C. Abnormal cholesterol metabolism
D. Abnormal calcium metabolism

60. **Best diagnostic method for Meckel's diverticulum is : TN 1996, 98**
A. Barium study
B. Tc99 scan
C. Tc99 pertechnetium scan
D. Endoscopy

61. **A diffuse reduction in activity throughout the liver on a technetium 99m colloid scan can be seen in the following except : DNB 1989**
A. Lymphoma B. Portal vein thrombosis
C. Myelosclerosis D. Amoebic abscess
E. Budd-Chiari syndrome

62. **The best view to visualize minimum pneumoperitoneum is : Delhi 1981**
A. AP view of abdomen
B. Erect film of abdomen
C. Right lateral decubitus with horizontal beam
D. Left lateral decubitus with horizontal beam

63. **Narrow rigid and smooth bowel is seen in all except : DNB 1989**
A. Mesenteritis B. Panniculitis
C. Lymphosarcoma D. Tuberculosis
E. Tumour metastasis

64. **Liver metastasis from G.I. tract can sonographically present as : PGI 1981**
A. Highly Echogenic
B. Less Echogenic
C. Hypoechoic
D. Diffuse distortion of liver parenchyma

65. **Emphysematous cholecystitis is found mainly in patient with : AIIMS 1984**
A. Gout
B. Stone impacted in cystic duct
C. Poorly controlled diabetes
D. Arteriosclerotic disease

66. **'Coffe bean' sign indicates : AIIMS 1984**
A. Toxic megacolon.
B. Volvulus of caecum.
C. Strangulation of incompletely obstructed loop of small bowel.
D. Mesenteric artery embolism.

67. **Bull eye lesion in the barium meal is seen in : UP 1998**
A. Malignant melanoma
B. Carcinoma of lung
C. Leomyosarcoma
D. Metastatic tumour of breast

68. **Hepatosplenomegaly is seen in the following conditions except : Bihar 1989**
A. Histocytosis-X B. Myelosclerosis
C. Coeliac disease D. Kala-azar
E. Thalassaemia

69. **Best investigation of air in peritoneal cavity is : CMC 1998**
A. USS
B. Laprotomy
C. Laproscopy
D. X-ray abdomen erect new
E. CT Scan

Ans. 53. A 54. E 55. C 56. C 57. B 58. D 59. B 60. C 61. D 62. D
63. D 64. A 65. C 66. C 67. C 68. C 69. D

70. **Causes of bile-stained vomiting in neonate are all except : AIIMS 1985**
A. Meconium plug
B. Septicaemia
C. Choledochal cyst
D. Hirschsprung's disease
E. Malrotation of the bowel

71. **Gas within biliary tree can be seen on the plain abdominal radiograph in all except : PGI 1988**
A. Mesenteric infarction.
B. Patients who have had sphincterotomy of the lower end of the common bile duct.
C. Gallstone ileus.
D. Amoebic abscess.

72. **A pathognomonic X-ray sign of chronic pancreatitis is : AIIMS 1984**
A. Air under diaphragm
B. Sentinal loop
C. Widening of duodenal loop
D. Pancreatic calcification

73. **On renal ultrasound examination the cortical echo pattern increased compared to adjacent liver-spleen echo pattern in all ecept : AIIMS 1981**
A. Diabetes
B. Renal transplant rejection
C. Lymphoma
D. Chronic glomerulonephritis
E. Sarcoidosis

74. **True about Meckel's diverticula except : AIIMS 1983**
A. Occur in about 2% of the population.
B. Sometimes contain calculi.
C. Are rarely demonstrated on a small bowel meal.
D. Will usually demonstrated by a technetium 99 m colloid scan.
E. Are associated with accessory splenuculi.

75. **For pancreas, least invasive procedure is : Rajasthan 1998**
A. USG B. Endoscopy
C. Laparoscopy D. Laparotomy

76. **Ultrasonic appearance of hepatic hematoma is : AIIMS 1985**
A. Echogenic B. Isodence
C. Sonolucent D. All of the above

77. **Large intestinal obstruction will show all except : AIIMS 1982**
A. Dilated loops tend to be in the distribution of colon.
B. Haustral pattern is disturbed.
C. Colon has a 'cut off' sign at the side of obstruction.
D. Isolated loop distension with volvulus.

78. **Which is the rare and unreliable sign of appendicitis : Delhi 1983**
A. Appendix calculi
B. Widening of peritoneal fat line
C. Mass indenting the caecum
D. Gas in appendix
E. Blurring of peritoneal fat line

79. **String sign is seen in : AIIMS 1985; Kerala 1988; AI 1991**
A. Crohn's disease
B. TB of the ileocecal region
C. Idiopathic hypertrophic pyloric stenosis
D. All of the above

80. **In controlling oesophageal varicela bleeding, best results have been obtained with infusion of pitressin into : AMC 1983**
A. A peripheral vein
B. Coeliac artery
C. Superior mesenteric artery
D. Inferior mesenteric artery

81. **An ultrasound examination shows dilated intrahepatic biliary channels with a small gall bladder. The most likely diagnosis is : Karnataka 1994**
A. Gall bladder stone
B. Pancreatic calculus
C. Common bile duct stone
D. Ca head of Pancreas

82. **In a child, most common cause of abdominal mass with calcification is : PGI 1994**
A. Neuroblastoma B. Bladder stone
C. Wilm's tumor D. Pulm Koch's

83. **Neuroblastoma deposits in the liver known as : AP 1991**
A. Crigler Najjar syndrome
B. Rotor syndrome
C. Hutchinson syndrome
D. Pepper syndrome

84. **What percentage of patients of perforated peptic ulcer show free air under diaphragm : Rajasthan 1989, 90; DNB 1993**
A. 50 B. 75
C. 90 D. 100

85. **Free air under diaphragm is seen in the following except : Rajasthan 1991, 93**
A. Peritoneal dialysis
B. Bowel perforation
C. Immediate post-operative period
D. Uncomplicated intestinal obstruction

Ans. 70. C 71. A 72. D 73. C 74. D 75. A 76. D 77. B 78. D 79. D 80. C 81. C 82. A 83. D 84. B 85. D

86. A patient with obstructive jaundice and PT is 30 minutes, which investigation is contraindicated : Rajasthan 1992; MP 1994

A. PTC B. X-ray
C. CT Scan D. Ultrasound

87. Most radiosensitive part of GIT is : Rajasthan 1993

A. Oesophagus B. Stomach
C. Intestine D. Rectum

88. All the following are features of Splenic rupture except : TN 1999

A. Obliteration of Psoas shadow
B. Obliteration of splenic outline
C. Elevation of Left Diaphragm
D. Obliteration of Colonic Air Bubble

89. Pipe stem appearance of colon in X-ray is due to : PGI 1983, 86, 91; TN 1999

A. Early stage of ulcerative colitis
B. Late stage of ulcerative colitis
C. Crohn's disease
D. Amoebic colitis

90. Cholangiography via T-Tube done after how many days of cholecystectomy : TN 1999

A. 1- 5 days B. 5-9 days
C. 10-14 days D. 15-20 days

91. Rectal mucosa is damaged above : Kerala 1999

A. 1000 Rad B. 2000 Rad
C. 4000 Rad D. 6200 Rad

92. Double-bubble sign is seen is : AI 1994

A. Duodenal atresia B. Jejunal atresia
C. Ca stomach D. Gastric ulcer

93. On Ba Swallow, achalasia cardia appears as : AI 1994

A. Cork screw oesophagus
B. Generalized dilatation
C. Rat tail appearance
D. Generalized constriction

94. Invertogram for imperforate anus is done after : PGI 1998; Kerala 2001

A. 2 hrs B. 4 hrs
C. 6 hrs D. 8 hrs

95. In oral cholecystography GB not visualized, probable is : Rohtak 2001

A. Malabsorption
B. Gall bladder
C. Impaired hepatic function
D. All of the above

96. With reference to a patient having hematoma around spleen, consider the following signs in plain X-ray of abdomen : UPSC 2003

1. Obliteration of psoas shadow
2. Indentation of the left side of the gastric air bubble
3. Free fluid between gas filled intestinal coils
4. Evidence of pneumoperitoneum

Which of these are seen in the plain X-ray of abdomen in this case :

A. 1 and 2 B. 1 and 3
C. 1, 2 and 3 D. 2, 3 and 4

97. On radiography widened duodenal 'C' loop with irregular mucosal pattern on upper gastrointestinal barium series is most likely due to : AI 2004

A. Chronic pancreatitis
B. Carcinoma head of pancreas
C. Duodenal ulcer
D. Duodenal ileus

98. Worm like filling defect is seen in : COMEDK 2005

A. Erossive gastritis
B. Oesophageal varices
C. Carcinoma esophagus
D. Schatzki's ring

Ans.									
86. A	87. C	88. D	89. B	90. C	91. D	92. A	93. B	94. C	95. D
96. C	97. B	98. B							

EXPLANATIONS OF GIT

1. Ans.— C. Decreased splenic sequestration
2. Ans.— C. Demonstration of ulcer crate
3. Ans.— B. Duodenal ulcer
4. Ans.— A. Ultrasonography
5. Ans.— A. Valvulae conniventes
6. Ans.— C. Pneumoperitoneum
7. Ans.— D. Hypotonic
8. Ans.— B. Valvulae conniventes
9. Ans.— C. Technetium 99
10. Ans.— C. Increased transit time
11. Ans.— D. Diverticulum in esophagus
12. Ans.— C. CT scan
13. Ans.— C. Hirschsprungs disease
14. Ans.— C. Pancreas
15. Ans.— D. Splenic disease

    In Anatomical or functional asplenia there is no uptake of Tc labelled RBC's.
16. Ans.— B. Selective arteriography
17. Ans.— A. Peripheral location
18. Ans.— A. Raised hemidiaphragm
19. Ans.— A. Pancreas
20. Ans.— E. All are true
21. Ans.— C. Blunted costophrenic angle
22. Ans.— A. Acute pencreatitis
23. Ans.— B. Thinning of bowel wall
24. Ans.— C. Peristalsis remain undisturbed
25. Ans.— C. Both lateral umbilical ligament
26. Ans.— B. Gastrograffin
27. Ans.— B. Gas under hemidiaphragm
28. Ans.— C. Stomach displaced forwards
29. Ans.— D. Subphrenic abscess

    Pneumoperitoneum may be seen in trauma (penetrating or blunt injures), spontaneous causes (peptic or bowel perforation, toxic megacolon) and others (female genital tract lesions and pneumatosis intestinalis).
30. Ans.— D. Pneumatosis intestinalis
31. Ans.— C. Handek's niche
32. Ans.— B. Ulcus callosum
33. Ans.— A. Carman's sign
34. Ans.— B. USG
35. Ans.— B. Carcinoma head of pancreas

    Pancreatic metastasis may be seen in Melanoma, lung cancer, breast cancer, ovarian cancer, hepatocellular carcinoma, renal cell carcinoma and sarcoma.
36. Ans.— D. CT Scan
37. Ans.— A. Enteroclysis
38. Ans.— A. Volvulus of colon
39. Ans.— C. Brucellosis

    Splenic calcifications can be diseminated (phleboliths, granulomas due to histoplasmosis, TB, brucellosis), Capsular and parenchymal (pyogenic or tubercular, infarction, hematoma), Vascular (splenic artery calcification, splenic artery aneurysm, splenic infarcts), calcified cyst wall (congenital cyst, post-traumatic, echinococcal, cystic dermoid, epidermoid), generalized increased density (sickle cell anemia in 5%, hemachromatosis, thorotrast, lymphangiography). Mnemonic is HITCH (Histoplasmosis most common, infarcts (sickle cell), TB, cysts (echinococcal), haematoma).
40. Ans.— D. All of the above

41. Ans.— C. Intussusception

Coiled spring appearance is seen in anterograde and retrograde barium study. There may be beaklike abrupt narrowing of barium column demonstrating a central channel. On CT scan, there are multiple concentric rings (and three concentric cylinders). On USG, doughnut sign (on pseudokindey sign and on longitudinal section) are seen.

42. Ans.— C. Trauma

43. Ans.— C. A patent anus

44. Ans.— A. Boerhave syndrome

45. Ans.— E. On CT scan swelling confined to pancreatic head

46. Ans.— D. Ultrasonography

For OCG, bilirubin level should be below 5 mg%. IVC is preliminary investigation. Investigation of choice in obstructive Jaundice is ERCP.

47. Ans.— D. Any of the above

48. Ans.— A. CT

CT is also best for pancreatic neoplasms.

49. Ans.— C. Peritoneal dialysis

50. Ans.— D. Periampullary carcinoma of pancreas

51. Ans.— C. Coil spring appearence in Ba enema

52. Ans.— D. Vascular ectasia

53. Ans.— A. Gasric outlet obstruction

54. Ans.— E. Thalassaemia

55. Ans.— C. Within min. 3-4 8-9 Upto 12

56. Ans.— C. Characterless

57. Ans.— B. Ischemic colitis

58. Ans.— D. Bile composition

Dose used is 6 Tablets of 0.5 g 2 hours after evening meals. Bilirubin should be below 5 mg%. Absolutely contraindicated in serious liver disease and relatively contraindicated in peritonitis, postoperative ileus and acute pancreatitis.

59. Ans.— B. Hemolytic anemias

60. Ans.— C. Tc99 pertechnetium scan

61. Ans.— D. Amoebic abscess

62. Ans.— D. Left lateral decubitus with horizontal beam

63. Ans.— D. Tuberculosis

64. Ans.— A. Highly Echogenic

65. Ans.— C. Poorly controlled diabetes

66. Ans.— C. Strangulation of incompletely obstructed loop of small bowel.

67. Ans.— C. Leomyosarcoma

68. Ans.— C. Coeliac disease

69. Ans.— D. X-ray abdomen erect new

70. Ans.— C. Choledochal cyst

71. Ans.— A. Mesenteric infarction

72. Ans.— D. Pancreatic calcification

73. Ans.— C. Lymphoma

74. Ans.— D. Will usually demonstrated by a technetium 99m colloid scan.

75. Ans.— A. USG

76. Ans.— D. All of the above

77. Ans.— B. Haustral pattern is disturbed

78. Ans.— D. Gas in appendix

79. Ans.— D. All of the above

Other signs are terminal ileum involvement, discrete ulcers, cobblestoning, skip areas, mesenteric masses, fistulae and rarely duodenal or esophageal involvement.

80. Ans.— C. Superior mesenteric artery

81. Ans.— C. Common bile duct stone

82. Ans.— A. Neuroblastoma

83. Ans.— D. Pepper syndrome

84. Ans.— B. 75

85. Ans.— D. Uncomplicated intestinal obstruction

86. Ans.— A. PTC

87. Ans.— C. Intestine

88. Ans.— D. Obliteration of Colonic Air Bubble

89. Ans.— B. Late stage of ulcerative colitis

Also called Lead pipe colon (there is rigidity and symmetric narrowing of lumen).

90. Ans.— C. 10-14 days

91. Ans.— D. 6200 Rad

92. Ans.— A. Duodenal atresia

It is also seen in annular pancreas.

93. Ans.— B. Generalized dilatation

Rat tail appearance is seen in carcinoma stomach.

94. Ans.— C. 6 hrs

95. Ans.— D. All of the above

96. Ans.— C. 1, 2 and 3

Plain X-ray feature of late rupture of spleen

* Obliteration of splenic outline	* Obliteration of psoas shadow
* Indentation of the left side of the lower gastric air bubble	* Fracture of one or more ribs of the left side
* Elevation of left hemi-diaphragm	* Free fluid between gas filled intestinal coils

97. Ans.— B. Carcinoma head of pancreas

Barium meal X-ray of the upper GI tract will show some distortion of the pattern of gastric antrum and duodenum in Ca head of pancreas.

- **Sometimes the barium filled C of the duodenum will be widened in cancer head of the pancreas. This is known as "Pad" sign.**
- **Sometimes in periampullary carcinoma a filling defect may be seen in duodenum in the appearance of a reversed 3 (— sign).**

98. Ans.— B. Oesophageal varices.

Technelium-99m sulphur colloid is used for liver, spleen, bone marrow, acute rejection of renal transplant, lower GI bleeding, gastric emptying etc. Imaging is taken 15-30 min post I.V. injection.

5

IMPORTANT TEXT OF UROGENITAL SYSTEM

GENITOURINARY SYSTEM

RENAL MASS

Unilateral renal masses

Solid Masses

A. Tumors

a) Malignant : Adenocarcinoma, malignant lymphoma/Hodgkin disease, adult nephroblastoma, metastasis, Wilms tumor, sarcoma, oncocytoma, invasive transitional cell carcinoma

b) Benign: Adenoma, hamartoma (angiomyolipoma), mesenchymal tumor (lipoma, fibroma, myoma, **hemangioma).**

B. Inflammatory masses :

Acute focal bacterial nephritis, renal abscess, xanthogranulomatous pyelonephritis, malakoplakia, tuberculoma.

Fluid filled masses

A. Cysts

a) Simple renal cyst

b) Inherited cystic disease:

Multicystic dysplastic kidney disease (Potter Type-II), multilocular cystic nephroma.

c) Focal hydronephrosis

B. Arteriovenous malformation

Bilateral renal masses

A. *Tumors*

1. Malignant lymphome/Hodgkin disease
2. Metastasis
3. Bilateral malignant or benign renal tumors

B. *Cysts*

1. Adult polycystic kidney disease
2. Acquired cystic kidney disease

Renal mass in neonate

A. *Unilateral*

1. Multicystic kidney (15%)
2. Hydronephrosis (25%)
   a) UPJ obstruction
   b) Upper moiety of duplication
3. Renal vein thrombosis
4. Mesoblastic nephroma
5. Rare : Wilms tumor, Teratoma

B. *Bilateral*

1. Hydronephrosis
2. Polycystic kidney disease
3. Multicystic kidney + contralateral hydronephrosis
4. Nephroblastomatosis
5. Bilateral multicystic kidney

CORTICAL RIM NEPHROGRAM

= Rim of cortex continues to receive flow from capsular vessels.

Causes:

1. Acute total main renal artery occlusion
2. Renal vein thrombosis
3. Acute tubular necrosis
4. Severe chronic urinary obstruction

CALCIFIED RENAL MASS

A calcified renal mass is malignant in about 75% of cases

A. *Tumor*

1. Renal cell carcinomas calcify in 10%.
   * Calcifications generally non-peripheral, sometimes along fibrous capsule.
2. Wilms tumor

B. *Infection*

1. Abscess
   — Tuberculous abscess frequently calcifies.
   — Pyogenic abscess rarely calcifies.
2. Echinococcal cyst
   Renal involvement in 3% of hydatid disease; 50% of echinococcal cysts calcify.
3. Xanthogranulomatous pyelonephritis
   * Large obstructive calculus in >70%.

C. *Cysts*

Calcification related to prior hemorrhage and infection :

1. Simple renal cysts calcify in 1% .
2. Multicystic dysplastic kidney disease (in adult).
3. Adult polycystic kidney disease.
4. Milk of calcium (cyst, caliceal diverticulum, obstructed hydrocalyx).

D. *Dx: Residual pantopaque used in cyst puncture*

D. *Vascular*

1. Subcapsular/perirenal hematoma.
2. Renal artery aneurysm circular ***cracked egg-shell appearance.***
3. Congenital/post-traumatic arteriovenous fistula.

MALE GENITAL TRACT

Calcifications of male genital tract :

A. *Vas Deferens*

1. Diabetes melitus : In muscular outer layer
2. Degenerative changes
3. TB, syphilis, non-specific UTI: intraluminal

B. *Seminal Vesicles*

Gonorrhea, TB, schistosomiasis, bilharziosis

C. *Prostate*

Calcified corpora amylacea, TB

SCROTAL MASS

1.	Inflammation	48%
2.	Hydrocele	24%
3.	Torsion	9%
4.	Varicocele	7%
5.	Spermatocele	4%
6.	Cysts	4%
7.	Malignant tumor	2%
8.	Benign tumour	0.7%

MCQ's OF UROGENITAL SYSTEM

What is important in Urogenital System

Peritoneum (Ascites), Polycystic/Horseshoe kidney, Hydronephrosis, TB, Flea beaten kidney, White enlarged kidney, Renal Atrophy, Renal Calculi, Bladder (Calculi, Diverticuli, Carcinoma), Adrenal (Calcification, Tumours), Male Genital Tract (Testicular masses, Tumours, Calcification), Female Genital Tract (Ovarian, Uterine and Cervix, Infertility, Estimation of foetal maturity), Pregnancy

1. **Finding of a "beaded appearance of vas deferens during a vesiculogram indicates : Delhi 1986, 90**
   A. Gonorrhoea B. Tuberculosis
   C. Non-specific infection D. Bilharziasis
2. **The earliest change of chronic pylonephritis may be : Delhi 1985, 86, 92**
   A. Cortical retraction
   B. Crowding of major calyces
   C. Increased forniceal angle
   D. Dilatation of pelvis
3. **Multiple uretheral strictures are almost diagnostic of : AIIMS 1982, 89, 90**
   A. Retroperitoneal fibrosis
   B. Tuberculosis
   C. Retroperitoneal abscess
   D. Schistosomiasis
4. **Normal GRF on first day of life is about——— % of adult values : DNB 1992, 96**
   A. 13 B. 21
   C. 44 D. 60
5. **Commonest cause of bladder wall calcification with relatively normal distensibility is : AIIMS 1985**
   A. Post-irradiation B. Tuberculosis
   C. Schistosomiasis D. Leiomyosarcoma
6. **Which of the following is most useful in distinguishing a renal cyst from a renal carcinoma : PGI 1982, 89**
   A. Intravenous urogram
   B. Retrograde pyelogram
   C. Radio-active venogram
   D. Renal Arteriogram
7. **Average Scrotal wall thickness is —— mm : AIIMS 1985, 94**
   A. 3—6 B. 9—145
   C. 18—25 D. 25—35
8. **In renal tuberculosis angiography is of value in order to : Delhi 1985**
   A. Show the extent of parenchymal involvement
   B. Establish the Diagnosis
   C. Both A and B
   D. None of the above
9. **A young man with tuberculosis presents with massive recurrent hemoptysis. For angiographic treatment which vascular structure should be evaluated first : AIIMS 2002**
   A. Pulmonary artery B. Bronchial artery
   C. Pulmonary vein D. Superior vena cava
10. **Cortical rim nephrogram is seen in following except : DNB 1990**
    A. Acute tubular necrosis
    B. Urinary obstruction
    C. Renal vein thrombosis
    D. Acute total main renal artery occlusion

Match the following (Ques 11 to 15) :
A. Stein leventhal Syndrome
B. Serous cystadenoma
C. Mucinous cystadenoma
D. Cystosarcoma botyroides
E. Hydatidiform mole

11. **Amniographic appearance are characteristic revealing multiple small rounded radiolucencies.**
12. **Multiloculated invasive mass due to multiple polypoidal instrusions is seen.**
13. **Multiloculated tumors are mostly unilateral and benign.**
14. **Psammomatous calcification in parent and metastatic tumours when present is diagnostic of this disease.**
15. **Pelvic Pneumogram reveals smooth enlarged ovaries, disproportionately large in relation to uterus.**

Ans.	1. B	2. C	3. B	4. B	5. C	6. D	7. A	8. A	9. B	10. B
	11. E	12. D	13. C	14. B	15. A					

16. Radiological diagnosis of pregnancy can be made at : Karnataka 1989

A. 12 weeks gestation B. 16 weeks gestation
C. 20 weeks gestation D. 24 weeks gestation

17. Radio opaque shadow is seen in the following ovarian tumour : Karnataka 1989

A. Simple serous cyst B. Granulosa cell tumour
C. Dermoid D. Muscinous cystadenoma

Match the following (Ques. 18 to 21) : AIIMS 1984

A. Bilateral renal cortical necrosis
B. Chronic glomerulonephritis
C. Medullary cystic disease
D. Medullary sponge kidney
E. Renal tubular acidosis

18. Small kidneys with diffuse granular cortical calcification.

19. Tramway (double line) calcification is characteristic radiographic finding.

20. Hepatic fibrosis and dilated bile ducts may be associated with the disease.

21. Radiographically presents as diffuse nephrocalcinosis with staghorn.

22. "Champagne glass" pelvis is seen in : AMU 1987

A. Achondroplasia
B. Cretinism
C. Down's syndrome
D. Congenital dislocation of hip

23. The most serious complication of percutaneous antegrade pyelography is : AIIMS 1989

A. Bleeding
B. Excessive pressure with extravasation
C. Introduction of infection
D. Clot obstructions
E. Puncture of adjacent organs

24. Commonest cause of renovascular hypertension is : DNB 1990

A. Fibromuscular dysplasia
B. Neoplasm
C. Renal cysts
D. Atherosclerosis

25. The best initial treatment for ureteric calculus above pelvic brium is : AI 1995

A. Antibiotics and diuretics
B. Diuretics only
C. Lithotripsy
D. Pyelolithotomy

26. USG and radionucleide are used in : Orissa 1998

A. Renal trauma
B. Renovascular HT
C. Renal parenchymal disease
D. Renal TB

27. In a case of ARF with total anuria, USG was found to be normal. Next live of inv. is : AI 1999

A. Retrograde pyelography
B. IVP
C. Anterograde pyelography
D. DTPA renogram

28. In urinary Schistosomiasis, calcification is commonly seen in : Rohtak 1986

A. Bladder
B. Entire Ureter
C. Lower half the ureters
D. Upper half of the ureters

29. Simplest diagnostic aid to differentiate a solid & cystic renal cyst is : TN 1996

A. USG B. CT Scan
C. MRI D. Plain X-ray

30. The "String of beads" or sausage appearance of the renal artery is due to : PGI 1982

A. Fibromuscular hyperplasia
B. Sub-adventitial fibroplasia
C. Medial fibroplasia with aneurysms
D. Outercoat fibroplasia with aneurysms
E. None of the above

31. Bilateral enlarged kidneys can be seen in following except : BHU 1987

A. Diabetes mellitus B. Acute tubular necrosis
C. Acromegaly D. Cushing's syndrome
E. Multiple myeloma

32. In a nephroblastoma, following are true except : AIIMS 1986

A. Occurs in children under 5
B. Is associated with horseshoe kidney
C. Is bilateral in about 5% of cases
D. Metastasis most common to bone
E. Rarely calcifies

33. Exclude one which does not exhibit enlarged kidneys : PGI 1985

A. Polycystic kidneys B. Pyelonephritis
C. Leukaemias D. Amyloidosis

34. Hypertrophy of prostate manifests itself as : AMU 1984

A. Cystitis
B. Vesical diverticula
C. Elongation of posterior urethra
D. All are true

35. In a non-distended urinary bladder, wall thickness is below —— mm : AIIMS 1984

A. 1 B. 3
C. 5 D. 7

Ans.										
	16. B	17. C	18. B	19. A	20. D	21. E	22. A	23. A	24. D	25. A
	26. B	27. D	28. A	29. A	30. C	31. D	32. D	33. B	34. D	35. C

36. Lightwood syndrome is a variant of : DNB 1989
A. Post. urethral valves
B. Hemolytic uremic syndrome
C. Renal tubular acidosis, proximal type
D. Renal tubular acidosis, distal type

37. Renal angle is a point which corresponds to the junction of : Rohtak 1990
A. 10th rib and lateral border of sacrospinalis
B. 10th rib and medial border of the sacrospinalis
C. 12th rib and lateral border of the sacrospinalis
D. 12th rib and medial border of sacrospinalis

38. Deflection of renal axis suggests : DNB 1991
A. Wedging of vertebra
B. Retroperitoneal tumours
C. Duplicated kidneys
D. All of the above

39. 9 months old child with three episodes of UTI, investigation not to be done is : AI 1995
A. Cystoscopy B. Voiding urethrogram
C. Ultrasound D. Radionucleotide scan

40. Sonographic appearance of renal transplant rejection is : AMU 1987
A. Increased echogenicity
B. Collection of fluid around kidney
C. Decrease in size of kidney
D. Increased kidney size

41. Psammomatous-like calcification seen in suprapubic region of a male pelvis may be seen in presence of : DNB 1991
A. Calculus
B. Bladder diverticula
C. Bladder neoplasm
D. Tuberculous seminal vesiculitis

42. Renal scan should be done with ——— position : AMU 1990
A. Supine B. Prone
C. Sitting D. Left lateral

43. In a child a filling defect in the bladder at intravenous urography can be due to : UPSC 1983
A. Rhabdomy sarcoma
B. A phaeochromocytoma
C. An ectopic ureterocele
D. Posterior urethral valves
E. Schistosoma infection

44. Following are Radiosensitive tumours except : AIIMS 1997
A. Melanoma B. Osteosarcoma
C. Lymphoma D. Ewings sarcoma

45. Localisation of placenta at 34 weeks of pregnancy is best done by : AMU 1986
A. Auscultation of uterine souffle
B. Plain X-ray abdomen
C. Ultrasonography
D. Soft tissue placentography

46. Suprarenal calcification can occur in the following except : AMU 1985
A. Phaeochromocytoma
B. Wokman's disease
C. Idiopathic hypercalcaemic syndrome
D. Conn's syndrome
E. Histoplasmosis

47. In nephrogram, dye is seen in : Delhi 1993, 95, 96
A. PCT B. DCT
C. CT D. Capillaries

48. The treatment of choice of stage-IIIB carcinoma of the uterine cervix is : DNB 1991
A. Surgery
B. Chemotherapy
C. Radiotherapy
D. Surgery followed by chemotherapy

49. Rim's sign on IVP is seen in : PGI 1998
A. Massive hydronephrosis
B. Polycystic ovary
C. Polycystic kidney
D. Ectopic ureter

50. Gestational age in third trimester is assessed by ultrasound of the following : AMU 1986
A. Length of femur B. Length of foetus
C. Biperietal D. Size of placenta

51. Estimation of feotal maturity by biparietal sonic measurement is accurate to within —— : AIIMS 1987
A. 3 - 7 days B. 7- 10 days
C. 10 - 15 days D. 14 - 20 days
E. 3 - 4 weeks

52. The immunosuppressent of the choice in Renal transplant is : JIPMER 1992
A. Azathioprine B. Hydroxyurea
C. Cyclophosphamide D. Steroid

53. Point B in the treatment of Ca. Cervix by radiotherapy corresponds to : AIIMS 1992
A. Obturator nodes B. MacKenrodts ligaments
C. Ischial tuberosity D. Round ligaments

54. Bead cystogram is used for the diagnosis of : TN 1993
A. Ca. bladder B. Stress incontinence
C. Thimble bladder D. Diverticulam

Ans.									
36. C	37. C	38. D	39. D	40. D	41. C	42. B	43. D	44. A	45. C
46. C	47. D	48. C	49. A	50. A	51. B	52. A	53. A	54. B	

55. **In child bearing period in female, the abdominal X-ray should be taken : AI 1993**
A. 10 days after LMP
B. Last 10 days of cycle
C. Within 10 days of LMP
D. During the middle of the cycle

56. **MCU is not indicated in : AI 1993**
A. Recurrent URI in a child
B. Suspected urethral valves
C. Renal mass
D. During the middle of the cycle

57. **'Calyceal cresent' seen on excretory urogram : PGI 1982, 87**
A. Due to distorted collecting tubules
B. Associated with elevated intrapelvic pressure
C. Indicated obstructive uropathy
D. All of the above

58. **Persistent nephrogram is seen in : Delhi 1988**
A. Ureteric obstruction B. Horseshoe kidney
C. Renal tumour D. Hydronephrosis

59. **Possible long term complication of the use of shock wave lithotripsy for renal calculi is : NIMHANS 1986**
A. Hemolytic units
B. Hypertension
C. Retroperitoneal fibrosis
D. Development of renal tumours

60. **The following are seen in a patient with chronic renal failure on haemodialysis except : PGI 1983, 89**
A. Abnormalities affecting the ulnar margins of the phalanges.
B. Markedly elevated alkaline phosphatase.
C. Sclerosis of vertebral end plates.
D. Metastatic calcification.
E. Periosteal new bone formation.

61. **Ultrasound and radionuclide studies are primary imaging modalities used for the assessment of : Orissa 1998**
A. Renal trauma
B. Renovascular hypertension
C. Renal tuberculosis
D. Renal transplant

62. **In a renal cell Ca., IF IVC and renal vein blocked with thrombosia, diagnosis is made by : AIIMS 1999**
A. Colour doppler B. IVP
C. USG D. CT Scan

63. **All the following are true about angiomyolipomas of kidneys except : Kerala 2000**
A. Ultrasound is the investigation of choice
B. It is associated with tuberous sclerosis
C. It is considered a hamartoma
D. It may present with flank pain
E. Angiography may reveal aneurysms

64. **'Thimble' bladder is seen in : AI 1991**
A. Cystitis cystica
B. Chronic tubercular cystitis
C. Neurogenic bladder
D. Acute tubercular cystitis

65. **Commonest cause of bilateral spider leg deformity of calyces seen on excretory urography is : DNB 1990; AI 1991**
A. Hypernephroma B. Polycystic kidney
C. Hydronephrosis D. Wilm's tumour

66. **Testicular tumors occur frequently in : DNB 1990; AI 1991**
A. Testis with scrotal hernia
B. Undescended abdominal testis
C. Mumbs orchitis
D. Following injury to testis

67. **All are related to development of bladder cancer except : AI 1991**
A. Tuberculosis B. Bilharziasis
C. Aniline dyes D. Chronic irritation

68. **Snow storm appearance is seen in USG of : AI 2001**
A. Hydatidiform mole B. Ectopic pregnancy
C. Twins D. IUD

69. **A dense persistent nephrogram may be seen in all of the following except : AIIMS 2002**
A. Acute ureteral obstruction
B. Systemic hypertension
C. Severe hypertension
D. Dehydration

70. **Which of the following imaging modality is most sensitive to detect early renal tuberculosis : AIIMS 2002**
A. Intravenous urography
B. Ultrasound
C. Computed tomography
D. Magnetic resonance imaging

71. **Choice of adjuvant treatment for endometrial carcinoma stage-IA, grade-I is: AI 2004**
A. Radiotherapy
B. Chemotherapy
C. Chemotherapy plus radiotherapy
D. No treatment

72. **Adrenal adenoma on CT which is not true : AI 2009**
A. Hypodense mass
B. Micro-calcification can be present
C. Contrast appears early and washes out late
D. Regular border

73. **Papillary necrosis features are all except : AIIMS 2009**
A. Egg in cup
B. Hyperdense nephrogram
C. Calyceal horns
D. "Ring shadows"

Ans.										
	55. C	56. C	57. D	58. C	59. B	60. A	61. D	62. A	63. A	64. D
	65. B	66. B	67. A	68. A	69. B	70. A	71. D	72. C	73. B	

EXPLANATIONS OF UROGENITAL SYSTEM

1. Ans.— B. Tuberculosis
2. Ans.— C. Increased forniceal angle
3. Ans.— B. Tuberculosis
4. Ans.— B. 21
5. Ans.— C. Schistosomiasis
6. Ans.— D. Renal Arteriogram
7. Ans.— A. 3—6
8. Ans.— A. Show the extent of parenchymal involvement
9. Ans.— B. Bronchial artery
10. Ans.— B. Urinary obstruction
11. Ans.— E. Hydatidiform mole
12. Ans.— D. Cystosarcoma botyroides
13. Ans.— C. Mucinous cystadenoma
14. Ans.— B. Serous cystadenoma
15. Ans.— A. Stein leventhal Syndrome
16. Ans.— B. 16 weeks gestation
17. Ans.— C. Dermoid

    Dermoid ovary on plain X-ray (diagnostic in 40%) shows tooth or bone and fat density.
18. Ans.— B. Chronic glomerulonephritis
19. Ans.— A. Bilateral renal cortical necrosis
20. Ans.— D. Medullary sponge kidney
21. Ans.— E. Renal tubular acidosis
22. Ans.— A. Achondroplasia

    Champagne glass appearance is due to flattened iliac wings. Pelvis may also show rolling gout, square shaped flat non-inflated pelvic bones with tomb-stone configuration, decreased acetabular angle and small sacrosciatic notch.
23. Ans.— A. Bleeding
24. Ans.— D. Atherosclerosis
25. Ans.— A. Antibiotics and diuretics

    Micturating cystourethrogram is done to demonstrate urethra and bladder neck (in males) and to demonstrate bladder mechanisms in particular stress incontinence and in children, posterior urethral valves.
26. Ans.— B. Renovascular HT
27. Ans.— D. DTPA renogram

    The compound is fixed in the tubules with a low extraction rate and good images may be obtained 1-2 hours after injection.
28. Ans.— A. Bladder
29. Ans.— A. USG
30. Ans.— C. Medial fibroplasia with aneurysms
31. Ans.— D. Cushing's syndrome
32. Ans.— D. Metastasis most common to bone
33. Ans.— B. Pyelonephritis
34. Ans.— D. All are true
35. Ans.— C. 5
36. Ans.— C. Renal tubular acidosis, proximal type
37. Ans.— C. 12th rib and lateral border of the sacrospinalis
38. Ans.— D. All of the above
39. Ans.— D. Radionucleotide scan
40. Ans.— D. Increased kidney size
41. Ans.— C. Bladder neoplasm
42. Ans.— B. Prone
43. Ans.— D. Posterior urethral valves
44. Ans.— A. Melanoma

    RBC's are most resistant (Remember oxygenated cells are most resistant).
45. Ans.— C. Ultrasonography
46. Ans.— C. Idiopathic hypercalcaemic syndrome
47. Ans.— D. Capillaries
48. Ans.— C. Radiotherapy

49. Ans.— A. Massive hydronephrosis

50. Ans.— A. Length of femur

51. Ans.— B. 7- 10 days

52. Ans.— A. Azathioprine

53. Ans.— A. Obturator nodes

54. Ans.— B. Stress incontinence

55. Ans.— C. Within 10 days of LMP

56. Ans.— C. Renal mass

57. Ans.— D. All of the above

58. Ans.— C. Renal tumour

59. Ans.— B. Hypertension

60. Ans.— A. Abnormalities affecting the ulnar margins of the phalanges.

61. Ans.— D. Renal transplant

62. Ans.— A. Colour doppler

63. Ans.— A. Ultrasound is the investigation of choice

Angiomyolipoma is also called renal hamartoma (Tumor composed of thick walled blood vessels, smooth muscle and fat. It is isolated in 80% and with tuberous sclerosis in 20%. Plain X-ray shows fat lucency, CT shows fat density and USG shows intensely echogenic tumor. Angiography is best and shows hypervascular mass in 95%. Sunburst/ Whorled/Onion peel appearances and no AV shunting.

64. Ans.— D. Acute tubercular cystitis

Seen on cystography and is due to fibrosis resulting in reduced capacity.

65. Ans.— B. Polycystic kidney

In horse shoe kidney, there is flower-vase type and in poly-cystic kidney, horse-shoe shaped (due to stretched calyces over cysts) and in hydronephrosis there is dilatation of pelvis.

66. Ans.— B. Undescended abdominal testis

Seminoma is more common.

67. Ans.— A. Tuberculosis

It most often originates in mucous membrane and first suspicion of chemical cause was raised by Rehn (1894). The chemical recognized are β naphthylamine, benzidine, β-naphthylamine, auramine and magenta.

68. Ans.— A. Hydatidiform mole

Sonography of liver, kidneys and spleen is also carried out. It has to be differentiated from missed abortion or degenerated fibroid.

69. Ans.— B. Systemic hypertension

70. Ans.— A. Intravenous urography

71. Ans.— D. No treatment

72. Ans.— C. Contrast appears early and washes out late

73. Ans.— B. Hyperdense nephrogram

The papillary/caliceal abnormalities of renal papillary necrosis fall into two groups :

1. Characteristic of papillary necrosis—> tracks and horns from the calices, the 'egg in a cup' appearance, and ring shadows.
2. Non-specific findings—>clubbed, blunt, or trauncated calices.

Papillary Necrosis :

* The commonest cause of papillary necrosis is analgesic nephropathy. Analgesic mixtures containing phenacetin have been most commonly implicated.
* Other major cause of papillary necrosis are diabetes, sickle-cell nephropathy and obstruction with infection.
* The papilla is particularly sensitive to ischemia and this seems likely to be the common etiological factor whatever the precipitating cause.

6

IMPORTANT TEXT OF MUSCULOSKELETAL SYSTEM

METAPHYSEAL BEAKING

Normal (knees) in bowed legs
  Other causes of bowed legs
Epiphyseal metaphyseal fractures in normal bone and battered child syndrome
Blount disease
Epiphyseal metaphyseal fractures in Breech delivery
Rickets
Hyperparathyroidism
Neurologic dIsease
Leukemia, lymphoma
Metastatic disease
Osteomyelitis
Congenital infections
Metabolic bone disease (premature)
Menkes kinky hair syndrome
Scurvy (Pelkan spurs)
Hypophopharasia
Desbuquis syndrome

ENLARGED VERTEBRAL BODY

1. Paget vertebral body
   * "picture framing"; bone sclerosis
2. Gigantism
   * increase in height of body + disc
3. Myositis ossificans progressiva
   * bodies greater in height than width
   * osteoporosis
   * ossification of ligamentum nuchae

ENLARGED VERTEBRAL FORAMEN

1. Neurofibroma
2. Congenital absence/hypoplasia of pedicle
3. Dural ectasia (Marfan syndrome, Ehlers Danlos syndrome)
4. Metastatic destruction of pedicle

STRAIGHTENING OF ANTERIOR BORDER

1. Ankylosing spondylitis
2. Paget's disease
3. Psoriatic arthritis
4. Reiter's disease
5. Rheumatoid arthritis
6. Normal variant

ANTERIOR SCALLOPING OF VERTEBRAE

1. Aortic aneurysm
2. Lymphadenopathy
3. Tuberculosis
4. Multiple myeloma (paravertebral soft tissue mass)

POSTERIOR SCALLOPING OF VERTEBRAE

Mnemonic : "HAMENTS"

Hurler disease, Hydrocephalus
Achondroplasia, Acromegaly
Marfan's syndrome
Ehlers-Danlos syndrome
Tumor (meningioma, ependymoma)
Syringohydromyelia

SPINE OSSIFICATION

A. Syndesmophyte = Ossification of annulus fibrosus associated with : ankylosing spondylitis, ochronosis.

B. Osteophyte
   = Ossification of anterior longitudinal ligament, paravertebral soft tissues associated with : diffuse idiopathic skeletal hyperostosis.

C. Flowing anterior ossification
   = Ossification of disc, anterior longitudinal ligament, paravertebral soft tissues.

D. Paravertebral ossification
   Associated with : psoriatric arthritis, Reiter's disease.

BONE-WITHIN-BONE VERTEBRA

= *"Ghost vertebra"* following stressful event during vertebral growth phase in childhood.

1. Stress line of unknown cause
2. Leukemia
3. Heavy metal poisoning
4. Thorotrast injection
5. Rickets
6. Scurvy
7. Hypothyroidism
8. Hypoparathyroidism

Ivory vertebra

Mnemonic : *"My Only Sister Left Home On Friday Past"*

Myelosclerosis

Osteoblastic metastasis

Sickle-cell disease

Lymphoma

Hemangioma

Osteopetrosis

Fluorosis

Paget disease

MCQ's OF MUSCULOSKELETAL SYSTEM

What is important in Musculoskeletal System

Anatomy of bone, Estimation of age, Epiphyseal fusion, Osteolytic, Osteosclerotic secondaries, Tumours, Changes in Important Systemic Diseases

1. **Subperiosteal erosions of middle phalanges on the radial aspect is characteristic of : AMC 1985, 91, 97**
   A. Hypoparathroidism B. Hyperparathyroidism
   C. Hyperthyroidism D. Hypothyroidism
2. **In bone infarcts, all are true except : AP 1990**
   A. In dysbaric osteonecrosis are commonlyin juxtaarticular
   B. Occur in Gaucher's disease
   C. Occur in thalassaemia major
   D. Are often diaphyseal in sickle cell disease
   E. Are seen in acute pancreatitis
3. **Eccentric subarticular radiolucent lesion in ends of long bones is suggestive of : JIMPER 1992**
   A. Osteoclastoma B. Osteogenic sarcoma
   C. Aneurysmal bone cyst D. Osteoid osteoma
4. **Dead bone on X ray looks : TN 1993**
   A. Highly radio-opaque
   B. Radio-opaque
   C. Radiolucent
   D. Not seen
5. **All are features of Achondroplasia except : PGI 1983, 93**
   A. Short and wide bones
   B. Lumbar canal stenosis
   C. Square shaped iliac bones
   D. Flattening of vertebral body
6. **Which of the following is not a feature of Osteogenesis imperfecta : PGI 1981, 86**
   A. Thin and fragile bones B. Blue sclera
   C. Otosclerosis D. Metaphyseal fracture
7. **The number of carpal bones seen in a radiograph of an infant is : PGI 1986, 94**
   A. 0 B. 2
   C. 3 D. 5
   E. 6
8. **Bone within bone vertebra may be seen in following except : PGI 1986**
   A. Rickets B. Scurvy
   C. Hypothyroidism D. Hypoparathyroidism
   E. Sickle cell anemia
9. **Age determination of a 18-years old on X-ray can be done from: Delhi 1994**
   A. Wrist B. Ankle
   C. Knee D. Shoulder
10. **Widespread patchy sclerosis of the skeleton can be seen in except : PGI 1983**
    A. Mast cell reticulosis
    B. Carcinoma of the breast
    C. Neuroblastoma
    D. Fluorosis
    E. Myeloid metaplasia
11. **Radiostrontium bone scans have been found positive in : AIIMS 1983**
    A. Fracture B. Bone tumours
    C. Paget's disease D. All are true
12. **Finding the non-union of the mandibular halves and of the zygomatic arches suggests : PGI 1981**
    A. Arachnoidactyly
    B. Cleidocranial dysostosis
    C. Osteogenesis imperfecta
    D. Morquio's disease
13. **X-ray examination in 'pulled elbow' usually shows : AIIMS 1984**
    A. Dislocation
    B. Subluxation
    C. Radial head fracture
    D. No osseous abnormality
14. **Onion peel appearance is seen in : NIMHANS 1986**
    A. Osteoclastoma B. Chondrosarcoma
    C. Osteosarcoma D. Ewing's sarcoma

Ans. 1. B 2. A 3. C 4. A 5. D 6. D 7. A 8. E 9. A 10. C
11. D 12. B 13. D 14. D

15. **Osteoporosis is diagnosed by all except :** **PGI 1989; AI 1996**
A. Ultrasonography B. CT Scan
C. Radiogammametry D. Plain X-ray

16. **Lytic lesion in upper end of tibia is expansile and has soap-buble appearance :** **AIIMS 1995**
A. Osteoclastoma B. Osteogenic Sarcoma
C. Ewing's Sarcoma D. Osteoblastoma

17. **Bifid manubrium may be seen in :** **DNB 1990**
A. Marfan's syndrome B. Down's syndrome
C. Achondroplasia D. TOF

18. **Picture frame vertebrae are seen typically in :** **AIIMS 1982**
A. Paget's disease B. Fluorosis
C. Ankylosing spondylitis D. Achondroplasia

19. **In Down's syndrome there are ------ ribs :** **Rohtak 1985**
A. 16 B. 18
C. 20 D. 22

20. **Rain drop lesions are seen in :** **AMU 1986**
A. Scurvy B. Thallasemia
C. Multiple myeloma D. Rickets

21. **Definite widening of the joints of hands and spine indicate :** **AIIMS 1981**
A. Gout B. Acromegaly
C. Hemophila D. Scleroderma

22. **X-ray appearance of avascular necrosis before appearance of typical features :** **PGI 1994**
A. Epiphyseal widening
B. Increase in joint line
C. Swelling of joint capsule
D. Fixed deformity

23. **In Madeling deformity cardinal abnormality is :** **AMU 1982**
A. Polydactyly
B. Congenital absence of ulna
C. Defective development of epiphysis of lower end of radius
D. Synostosis of radius and ulna

24. **Periosteal reactions are not seen in :** **AIIMS 1986**
A. Multiple myeloma
B. Actinomycosis
C. Infantile cortical hyperostosis
D. Osteoid osteoma
E. Syphilis

25. **The femur is fractured at birth at :** **Rajasthan 1993**
A. Upper one third B. Middle one third
C. Lower one third D. Neck region

26. **Both knee joints show narrowing, subarticular cystic defects and deep, wide inter condylar fossae indicating probable :** **AIIMS 1986**
A. Hemophilia B. Gout
C. Rheumatoid arthritis D. Degenerative Arthritis

27. **The cervical spine of a young adult showing several fused small joints bilaterally with underdeveloped vertebral bodies sharing narrowed intervertebral discs indicates probable childhood:** **AIIMS 1984**
A. Trauma B. Septic arthritis
C. Neurotropic disease D. Still's disease

28. **Cystic bone lesions with precocious sexual development and irregular pigmentation of the back indicate :** **AIIMS 1981**
A. Gaucher's disease B. Neurofibromatosis
C. Albright's syndrome D. Ollier's disease

29. **Sacroliitis is seen in the following except :** **DNB 1991**
A. Whipple's disease B. Sarcoidosis
C. Reiter's syndrome D. Behcet's disease
E. Psoriasis

30. **Radiological evidence of secondaries in spine is evident when —— % of bone has been destroyed :** **DNB 1993**
A. 10 B. 30
C. 50 D. 80

31. **Not characteristic of Brodie's abscess is :** **UPSC 1980**
A. Epiphyseal location
B. Sclerotic border
C. Chronic course
D. Localized radiant abscess in bone

32. **A multicystic process without bone reaction in the metaphysis of a long bone of a child is most likely:** **AIIMS 1982**
A. Bone infarct B. Tuberculosis
C. Osteogenesic sarcoma D. Pyogenic osteomyelitis

33. **Radiologically appreciable earliest sign of osteomyelitis is:** **AIIMS 1984**
A. Loss of muscle and fat planes
B. Periosteal reaction
C. Callus formation
D. Presence of sequestrum

34. **Increased density in the metaphyses of the long bones in children occurs in all except :** **AIIMS 1988**
A. Scurvy B. Syphilis
C. Mercury poisoning D. Caffey's disease
E. Metaphyseal dysostosis

35. **Osteoblastic metastasis is most frequently seen in malignancy of :** **AMU 1986; AI 1989**
A. Lung B. Liver
C. Kidney D. Prostate

Ans. **15. A** **16. A** **17. B** **18. A** **19. D** **20. C** **21. B** **22. A** **23. C** **24. A** **25. A** **26. A** **27. D** **28. C** **29. B** **30. C** **31. A** **32. B** **33. B** **34. D** **35. D**

36. All of the following causes increased bone density except : PGI 1980

A. Fluorosis B. Osteopetrosis
C. Cushing's syndrome D. Prostate metastasis

37. All of the following has decreased bone density except for : AIIMS 1980

A. Hypophosphatasia B. Steroid therapy
C. Osteomalacia D. Hypervitaminosis-A

38. Multiple Wormian bones can be seen in all except : AMU 1986

A. Neonatal hypothyroidism
B. Down's syndrome
C. Fibrous dysplasia
D. Progeria
E. Normal babies

39. Incorrect about pathological fractures : AMU 1986

A. Are commonly transverse in long bones.
B. In Paget's disease, commonly occurs in the shaft of the femur.
C. Commonly occur in the areas of chronic osteomyelitis.
D. Occur in the subtrochanteric region of the femoral shaft.
E. Occur as separation of the proximal femoral. epiphysis in children with renal osteodystrophy.

40. Earliest bone metastasis can be detected by : Karnataka 1994

A. Compound tomography
B. Plain X-rays
C. Radio-isoscope bone scan
D. Tomography

41. The best X- ray view for the evaluation of a scaphoid fracture is :

A. Anteroposterior B. Lateral
C. Oblique D. Axial

42. "Tumbling blocks " appearance in an X-ray of the spine is seen in : Karnataka 1994

A. Sickle cell disease B. Neurosyphilis
C. Multiple myeloma D. Ankylosing spondylitis

43. In trisomy 18 syndrome, all are true except : AIIMS 1986

A. Hypoplastic ribs are typical
B. The acetabular roof is flat
C. The first metacarpal is short
D. There is lumbar kyphoscoliosis
E. 'Rocker bottom' feet are characteristic

44. Jaccoud's arthritis occurs after the subsidence of severe bounds of : AIIMS 1985

A. Rheumatic fever
B. Crohn's disease
C. Amoebic colitis
D. Acute glomerulonephritis
E. Ulcerative colitis

45. Ossification may be commonly seen in ------- and ------. TN 1989

A. Mitral stenosis, lung bases
B. Mitral stenosis, lung apices
C. Mitral regurgitation, heart
D. Eisenmenger's complex, heart

46. Looser's zone, osteosclerosis and subperiosteal erosion are seen in : AIIMS 1997

A. Osteomalacia B. Renal osteodystrophy
C. Hyperparathyroidism D. Osteoporosis

47. The bone most commonly involved in osteoarthritic change of the knee joint is : AP 1989

A. Femur
B. Patella
C. Fibula
D. All are involved at the same time

48. A break in the Shenton's line is seen in : TN 1991

A. Down's syndrome
B. Congenital dislocation of hip
C. Cretinism
D. All of the above

49. The break in spondylosis is at the : AP 1989

A. Superior articular process
B. Inferior articular process
C. Spinous process
D. Pars interarticularis

50. Rib notching is seen in : AI 1989, 98

A. Coarctation of aorta
B. Neurofibromatosis
C. Following Blalock-Taussig operation
D. All of the above

51. Marginal posterior fracture passing through the radial articular surface is : AIIMS 1987

A. Smith's fracture B. Barton's fracture
C. Bennett's fracture D. Monteggia's fracture

52. Acro-osteolysis resorption of tips of the finger and toes is seen in : AIIMS 1990

A. Scleroderma B. Pyknodysostosis
C. Psoriasis D. All of the above

53. Which of the following does not describe chondroblastoma : AP 1990

A. Non-calcifying
B. Eccentric
C. Epiphyseal location
D. Simulates giant cell tumour of bone

54. When a growing bone is traumatised there may be a: TN 1990

A. Outward depression of epiphysis
B. Shaftward depression of epiphysis
C. Shaft ward depression of metaphysis
D. All of the above

Ans.										
	36. C	37. D	38. C	39. C	40. C	41. C	42. C	43. B	44. A	45. A
	46. B	47. B	48. B	49. D	50. D	51. B	52. D	53. A	54. C	

55. **"Umbau Zones" are in all except : AP 1990**
A. Osteomalacia
B. Rickets
C. Osteogenesis inperfecta
D. Osteomyelitis

56. **When fatigue fractures are multiple and symmetrical, the condition is known as : Kerala 1990**
A. Wax drippings B. Milkman's syndrome
C. Bone pearls D. None of the above

57. **The Roentgen criteria for sesamoid fractures are all the following except : Kerala 1990**
A. Irregular serrated line of division
B. Interrupted peripheral cortex
C. Multiplicity of fragments
D. Usual position

58. **Commonest cause of punched out lesions in phalanges is : Delhi 1998**
A. Enchondroma B. Chondrosarcoma
C. Aneurysmal bone cyst D. Multiple myeloma

59. **Calcification of the intervertebral disc is present in : Delhi 1998; AI 2000**
A. Maple syrup urine disease
B. Homocystinuria
C. Ankylosing spondylitis
D. Achondroplasia

60. **Sun-rays appearance is seen in following except : AI 1991; AIIMS 1998**
A. Multiple myeloma
B. Sturge-Weber syndrome
C. Osteogenic sarcomas
D. Meningioma

61. **Maisonneuve's sign indicates : AIIMS 1986, 97**
A. Clavicle fracture
B. Colles fracture
C. Smith fracture
D. Legg Calve Perthes disease

62. **Paget's disease of bone may be complicated by the following except : DNB 1989**
A. Banana fracture
B. Pseudofracture
C. Basilar invigination
D. Severe neurological complications
E. Strengthening of bone as a result of periosteal addition

63. **Impacted fracture is found in : Rajasthan 1993: DNB 1994**
A. Neck of femur B. Neck of humerus
C. Lower end of radius D. All of the above

64. **Transverse process fracture of spine most often occurs at ----- region. DNB 1992**
A. Cervical B. Dorsal
C. Lumbar D. Sacral

65. **Cone shaped epiphyses in the phalanges can be seen in the following except : BHU 1985**
A. After frost bite
B. As a normal variant
C. In cleidocranial dysostosis
D. In osteogenesis imperfecta

66. **Commonest site of spinal bifida is : AIIMS 1981**
A. Cervical B. Dorsal
C. Lumbar D. Sacral

67. **"Candle wax" appearance is seen in : Delhi 1983**
A. Osteogenesis imperfecta
B. Melorheostosis
C. Diaphyseal dysplasia
D. Exostosis

68. **Radiologically appreciable earliest sign of osteomyelitis is : AMU 1989**
A. Loss of muscles and fat planes
B. Periosteal reaction
C. Callus formation
D. Presence of sequestrum

69. **Commonest site of fracture in osteogenesis imperfecta is : DNB 1990**
A. Epiphysis B. Metaphysis
C. Diaphysis D. All of the above

70. **All the following statements are true about Fibrous Dysplasia except for : AMU 1986**
A. Ground-glass appearance of bone
B. Shepherd-Crook's appearance of femur
C. Commoner in females
D. Lesions are classically bilateral

71. **Normal metacarpal index is : DNB 1991**
A. Less than 5.4 B. 5.4 to 7.9
C. 8.4 to 10.4 D. More than 10.4

72. **Metacarpal index is increased in the case of : NIMHANS 1986**
A. Down's syndrome B. Marfan's syndrome
C. Turner's syndrome D. Jeene's disease

73. **Which of the following radio isotopes is used orally for treating a case of carcinoma presents with secondaries in bone : AIIMS 1997**
A. Strontium B. Co60
C. Cs D. Ra

74. **Earliest sign in Rheumatoid Arthritis is : Delhi 1995**
A. Decreased joint space
B. Periarticular Osteoporosis
C. Periarticular Soft Tissue Swelling
D. Reduced joint space

75. **'Fat pad sign' may be present in fracture of Lateral epicondyle of Salter type----injury. AIIMS 1997**
A. I B. II
C. III D. V

Ans.										
	55. C	56. B	57. D	58. A	59. C	60. B	61. B	62. E	63. C	64. C
	65. D	66. C	67. B	68. A	69. C	70. D	71. B	72. B	73. A	74. B
	75. B									

76. Avulsion fracture is most common in ------ metatarsal. **WB 1998**

A. I
B. II
C. III
D. IV

77. Early radiological sign of caries spine is : **DNB 1989**

A. Wedging of vertebra
B. Syndesmophyte formation
C. Formation of paravertebral abscess
D. Decreased joint space

78. Commonest type of spinal TB is : **NIMHANS 1989**

A. Anterior
B. Posterior
C. Central
D. Paradiscal
E. All

79. Radiological features of rickets are all except : **AIIMS 1984**

A. Narrowing and loss of zone of provisional calcification is earliest sign.
B. Metaphyseal margin becomes indistinct.
C. Frayed appearance.
D. Splaying and cupping of metaphyseal markings.
E. After one year of treatment only, recovery starts in X-rays.

80. In bony metastasis, primary should be looked for in all except : **PGI 1993**

A. Prostate
B. Thyroid
C. Stomach
D. Bronchus

81. Multiple osteolytic lesions in a 2 year child in skull and long bones are seen in : **PGI 1994**

A. Neuroblastoma
B. Histiocytosis
C. Thalassemia major
D. Wilms tumor

82. Flask shaped femur is seen in all except : **BHU 1985**

A. Osteomalacia
B. Osteopetrosis
C. Gaucher's disease
D. Thalassemia

83. Saw tooth metaphysis are seen in : **DNB 1991**

A. Acromegaly
B. Hyperparathyroidism
C. Congenital syphilis
D. Ochronosis

84. Syndactyly is seen in all of the following except : **PGI 1981**

A. Laurence Moon Biedel disease
B. Apert's syndrome
C. Trisomy - 13
D. Madelung deformity

85. Commonest fatal skeletal dysplasia of new-born is : **AIIMS 1981**

A. Osteogenesis imperfecta type-II
B. Thanatophoric dwarfism
C. Camptomelic dwarfism
D. Homozygos form of Achondroplasia

Match the X-ray land marks of foetal development with the period (Ques. 86 to 90): **AIIMS 1984**

A. 32 weeks
B. 36 weeks
C. 24 weeks
D. 12 weeks
E. 38 weeks

86. Distal femoral epiphysis

87. Foetal fat line

88. Calcaneous

89. Proximal tibial epiphysis

90. Spine and skull

91. Piano key sign is seen in : **Kerala 1999**

A. Osteoarthritis
B. Rheumatoid arthritis
C. Ankylosing spondylitis
D. Reiter's syndrome

92. In multiple myeloma, the radiologically differentiating manifestation is commonly seen in : **Kerala 1999**

A. Skull
B. Vertebra
C. Ribs
D. Pelvis

93. Splaying and cupping of the metaphysis is seen in : **Kerala 1999**

A. Rickets
B. Scurvy
C. Paget's disease
D. Lead poisoning

94. Radiological manifestation of acute osteomyelitis within first 8 days is : **TNPSC 1998**

A. Cystic swelling
B. Sequestrum
C. Subperiosteal new bone
D. Soft tissue swelling

95. Commonest cause of epiphyseal thickening in children is : **TNPSC 1998**

A. Congenital syphilis
B. Rickets
C. Scurvy
D. Osteo-chondrodystrophy

96. 76-years-old man presents with lytic lesions in the vertebra. X-ray skull showed multiple punched out lesions. The most likely diagnosis is : **AIIMS 2000**

A. Multiple myeloma
B. Hyperparathyroidism
C. Metastasis
D. Osteomalacia

97. Posterior iliac horn is seen in : **AIIMS 2002**

A. Nail patella syndrome
B. Ankylosing spondylitis
C. Hurler's syndrome
D. Marfan's syndrome

98. Chondrocalcinosis is seen in : **AIIMS 2002**

A. Hyperthyroidism
B. Ochronosis
C. Hypoparathyroidism
D. Hypervitaminosis-D

Ans.										
	76. D	77. D	78. D	79. E	80. C	81. A	82. A	83. C	84. B	85. B
	86. B	87. A	88. C	89. E	90. D	91. B	92. B	93. A	94. D	95. B
	96. A	97. A	98. B							

99. In bone scan, hot spots are seen in all except : JIPMER 2002

A. Osteoblastic metastasis
B. Multiple myeloma
C. Osteomyelitis
D. Bony lesions of hyperparathyroidism

100. Mutton-leg like gross appearance is seen in : CMC 2001

A. Osteosarcoma B. Osteoclastoma
C. Chondrosarcoma D. Ewing's sarcoma

101. Linear accelerator provide : A.P. 2002

A. Both electrons & X-rays
B. Only electrons
C. Protons
D. Electromagnetic rays

102. Which of the following is a recognized X-ray feature of Rheumatoid arthritis : AI 2003

A. Juxta-articular osteosclerosis
B. Sacrolitis
C. Bone-erosions
D. Peri-articular calcification

103. Fraying and cupping of metaphyses of long bones in an child does not occur in which of the following : AI 2003

A. Rickets
B. Lead poisoning
C. Metaphyseal dysplasia
D. Hypophosphatasia

104. The gold standard for the diagnosis of osteoporosis is : AI 2005

A. Dual energy X-ray absorptiometry
B. Single energy X-ray absorptiometry
C. Ultrasound
D. Quantitative computed tomography

105. Calcification of posterior spinal ligament is best diagnosed by : AI 2009

A. MRI B. CT
C. X-ray D. USG

106. Which of the following is not a cause of generalized increase in bone density in adult : Delhi 2009

A. Myelosclerosis B. Renal osteodystrophy
C. Fluorosis D. Caffey's diseases

Ans. **99. B** **100. A** **101. A** **102. C** **103. D** **104. A** **105. B** **106. D**

EXPLANATIONS OF MUSCULOSKELETAL SYSTEM

1. Ans.— B. Hyperparathyroidism
2. Ans.— A. In dysbaric osteonecrosis are commonly juxtaarticular
3. Ans.— C. Aneurysmal bone cyst
4. Ans.— A. Highly radio-opaque
5. Ans.— D. Flattening of vertebral body
6. Ans.— D. Metaphyseal fracture
7. Ans.— A. 0
8. Ans.— E. Sickle cell anemia
9. Ans.— A. Wrist
10. Ans.— C. Neuroblastoma
11. Ans.— D. All are true
12. Ans.— B. Cleidocranial dysostosis
13. Ans.— D. No osseous abnormality
14. Ans.— D. Ewing's sarcoma

    It occurs in middle of a long bone in childhood or adolescence. Radiography gives "cut onion" like appearance. Initial treatment is radiotherapy followed by amputation. Its origin is controversial whereas osteosarcoma is metaphyseal.
15. Ans.— A. Ultrasonography

    Osteoporosis is reduced bone mass of normal composition secondary to osteoclastic resorption (85%) or osteocytic resorption (15%). Serum Ca++ PO4 and Alkaline Phosphatase are normal.
16. Ans.— A. Osteoclastoma
17. Ans.— B. Down's syndrome
18. Ans.— A. Paget's disease
19. Ans.— D. 22
20. Ans.— C. Multiple myeloma
21. Ans.— B. Acromegaly
22. Ans.— A. Epiphyseal widening
23. Ans.— C. Defective development of epiphysis of lower end of radius.
24. Ans.— A. Multiple myeloma
25. Ans.— A. Upper one third
26. Ans.— A. Hemophilia
27. Ans.— D. Still's disease
28. Ans.— C. Albright's syndrome
29. Ans.— B. Sarcoidosis

    It is also typically seen in ankylosing spondylitis.
30. Ans.— C. 50
31. Ans.— A. Epyphyseal location

    It is seen in chronic osteomyelitis.
32. Ans.— B. Tuberculosis
33. Ans.— B. Periosteal reaction
34. Ans.— D. Caffey's disease
35. Ans.— D. Prostate

    Osteosclerotic metastases may arise from breast, GIT, Carcinoid, medulloblastoma, bladder, osteosarcoma and lymphoma whereas lytic metastasis may originate from lung, breast, kidney, thyroid, Ewing's sarcoma and mixed pattern from breast or lung.
36. Ans.— C. Cushing's syndrome
37. Ans.— D. Hypervitaminosis-A
38. Ans.— C. Fibrous dysplasia
39. Ans.— C. Commonly occur in the areas of chronic osteomyelitis.
40. Ans.— C. Radio-isoscope bone scan
41. Ans.— C. Oblique
42. Ans.— C. Multiple myeloma
43. Ans.— B. The acetabular roof is flat
44. Ans.— A. Rheumatic fever
45. Ans.— A. Mitral stenosis, lung bases
46. Ans.— B. Renal osteodystrophy
47. Ans.— B. Patella
48. Ans.— B. Congenital dislocation of hip
49. Ans.— D. Pars interarticularis

50. Ans.— D. All of the above

Rib notching of inferior margin is seen in vascular lesions (coarctation, thrombosis, Blalock-Taussig shunt, PS, TOF, Aberrant pulmonary artery, AV fistula, SVC obstruction), neurogenic causes (Inter-costal neuroma, neurofibromatosis, Polymyositis, paraplegia) or Osseous lesions (Hyperparathyroidism (HPH) Thalassemia, Melnick Needles syndrome). Rib notching on superior margin is seen in Rheumatoid arthritis, Scleroderma, SLE, HPH, Restrictive lung disease and Marfan's Syndrome.

51. Ans.— B. Barton's fracture

52. Ans.— D. All of the above

53. Ans.— A. Non-calcifying

54. Ans.— C. Shaft ward depression of metaphysis

55. Ans.— C. Osteogenesis inperfecta

56. Ans.— B. Milkman's syndrome

57. Ans.— D. Usual position

58. Ans.— A. Enchondroma

59. Ans.— C. Ankylosing spondylitis

Triad of degënerative arthritis, achronotic pigmentation and urine that turns black on alkalinization is characteristic of alkaptonuria. X-rays lumbar spine are virtually pathognomonic. They show degeneration and dense calcification of intervertebral discs and narrowing of intervertebral spaces.

60. Ans.— B. Sturge-Weber syndrome

'Soap bubble' appearance is in osteosarcoma and onion peel in. Ewing's tumor, Blow out distension in Aneurysmal done cyst and Honey comb in chronic osteomyelitis, osteoclastoma, Paget's disease and adamantinoma.

61. Ans.— B. Colles fracture

62. Ans.— E. Strengthening of bone as a result of periosteal addition.

63. Ans.— C. Lower end of radius

64. Ans.— C. Lumbar

65. Ans.— D. In osteogenesis imperfecta

66. Ans.— C. Lumbar

67. Ans.— B. Melorheostosis

68. Ans.— A. Loss of muscles and fat planes

69. Ans.— C. Diaphysis

70. Ans.— D. Lesions are classically bilateral

71. Ans.— B. 5.4 to 7.9

72. Ans.— B. Marfan's syndrome

73. Ans.— A. Strontium

74. Ans.— B. Periarticular Osteoporosis

75. Ans.— B. II

76. Ans.— D. IV

77. Ans.— D. Decreased joint space

Thoracolumbar spine is most often involved.

78. Ans.— D. Paradiscal

79. Ans.— E. After one year of treatment only, recovery starts in X-rays.

80. Ans.— C. Stomach

81. Ans.— A. Neuroblastoma

82. Ans.— A. Osteomalacia

83. Ans.— C. Congenital syphilis

84. Ans.— B. Apert's syndrome

85. Ans.— B. Thanatophoric dwarfism

86. Ans.— B. 36 weeks

87. Ans.— A. 32 weeks

88. Ans.— C. 24 weeks

89. Ans.— E. 38 weeks

90. Ans.— D. 12 weeks

91. Ans.— B. Rheumatoid arthritis

92. Ans.— B. Vertebra

Excretory urography should be cautiously done in multiple myeloma, proteinuria and diabetics with creatinine above 2 mg%.

93. Ans.— A. Rickets

94. Ans.— D. Soft tissue swelling

95. Ans.— B. Rickets

Hypothyroidism in a child also be associated with prolonged jaundice, decreased growth and mental retardation along with many other constitutional and systemic features. In epiphyseal dysgenesis bones involved are vertebrae, pelvis carpal and tarsal bones and epiphyses of tubular bones.

96. Ans.— A. Multiple myeloma

97. Ans.— A. Nail patella syndrome

98. Ans.— B. Ochronosis

99. Ans.— B. Multiple myeloma

100. Ans.— A. Osteosarcoma

101. Ans.— A. Both electrons & X-rays

102. Ans.— C. Bone-erosions

103. Ans.— D. Hypophosphatasia

104. Ans.— A. Dual energy X-ray absorptiometry

* Dual Energy X-ray absorptiometry (DEXA) can determine the density of any bone, is quite accurate and delivers negligible radiation.
* It is the gold standard for the diagnosis of osteoporosis
* Schwartz states :

  Osteoporosis is defined as a loss of bone per unit of volume. A more strict definition is bone with a bone mineral density (MBD) as measured by a dual energy X-ray absorptiometry (DEXA) scan of more than 2.5 cm below the norm.

105. Ans.— B. CT

Calcified posterior longitudinal ligament:

* Cervical spine involvement is most common.
* Likely to progress to myelopathy with canal compromise of 60% and sagittal canal diameter of 8 mm.
* Advanced cases of OPLL are easily recognized on routine radiography.
* Best evaluated with CT (for ossification) and MRI (for evaluation of cord).
* MRI is useful in assessing status of adjacent spinal cord.

106. Ans.— D. Caffey's diseases

7

MCQ's OF RADIATION PHYSICS & RADIOTHERAPY

What is important in Radiation Physics & Radiotherapy

Radioisotopes (Common ones, half lives, specific indications), Effects of radiations, Specific uses, Techniques and Adverse effects, Chemotherapy, Principles of Radiation Physics

1. **Cell most sensitive to radiation is : PGI 1984; Delhi 1991, 99**
   A. Lymphocyte B. Neutrophil
   C. Basophil D. Platelets
2. **Radioactivity was discovered by : AIIMS 1983**
   A. Marie Curie B. Pierre Curie
   C. Rutherford D. Eurico Formi
   E. Henri Bacquerol
3. **For a chest X-ray, patient is exposed to radiation of : Rohtak 1985**
   A. 1 rad B. 2 rads
   C. 3 rads D. 4 rads
   E. 5 rads
4. **Radiosensitising substances include : BHU 1985**
   A. Oxygen B. S R 2508
   C. Metronidazole D. Misonidazole
   E. All of the above
5. **Air is used in ionization chamber because it, except : AIIMS 1986**
   A. Is readily available
   B. Has a constant composition
   C. Has a low density
   D. Has an effective atomic number similar to that of soft tissue
6. **Radium emits : AIIMS 1986, 91, 97**
   A. Electrons B. X-rays
   C. Alpha D. Gamma rays
7. **Medical thermography is based on the principle of man emitting : AMU 1986**
   A. X-rays B. Ultrasonic rays
   C. Infrared radiation D. Ultraviolet radiation
8. **Out of the following which is being most commonly used now-a-days to measure radiation exposure : PGI 1983**
   A. Thimble chamber
   B. Geiger Muller counter
   C. Scintillation counter
   D. Thermoluminescence dose meter
9. **While doing Renography, Hippuran (Ortho-iodohippurate) is attached to : PGI 1982**
   A. Iodine - 125 B. Iodine - 131
   C. Iodine - 132 D. Iodine - 113
10. **"Target angle" in a Tele-therapy X-ray tube is : AIIMS 1981**
    A. 17 deg B. 30 deg
    C. 45 deg D. 60 deg
11. **Craniospinal irradiation is indicated in : Rohtak 1986; UPSC 1987; AP 1993; AI 1997**
    A. Acute lymphatic leukaemia after remission
    B. Hodgking's disease stage-IV
    C. Cancer breast stage-IV
    D. Seminoma testis stage-I
12. **After load intracavitory radiation is used in : AMU 1985**
    A. Carcinoma Cervix B. Carcinoma of colon
    C. Amoebiasis D. Crohn's disease
13. **The most radiosensitive tissue is : Orissa 1991**
    A. Brain B. Bone marrow
    C. Thyroid D. Liver
14. **The least radiosensitive tissue is : AIIMS 1983, 86**
    A. Nervous tissue B. Bone
    C. Kidney D. Thyroid
15. **Type of radiation called primary is that which : PGI 1982**
    A. Is controlled by milli ampere seconds
    B. Is controlled and cut off by cones
    C. Emerges from the tube and reaches the patient
    D. Emerges from patient and reaches the film
16. **'Grid' is a device which is used for : AIIMS 1985**
    A. Reducing scattered radiation
    B. Reducing patient's exposure time
    C. Reducing the contrast of the X-ray
    D. All of the above

Ans. 1. A 2. E 3. E 4. E 5. C 6. D 7. C 8. D 9. B 10. B
11. A 12. A 13. B 14. A 15. C 16. A

17. The best chest radiographs are performed at : AIIMS 1985

A. 60 - 90 Kvp B. 90 - 120 Kvp
C. 120 - 150 Kvp D. 150 - 200 Kvp

18. Ultrasound waves are produced by means of a .....crystal. AIIMS 1989

A. Ferromagnetic B. Piezoelectric
C. Ferro electric D. Paramagnetic

19. NMR uses Gyromagnetic property of : AIIMS 1989

A. Electron B. Proton
C. Positron D. Neutron

20. Field strength used in NMR is : AI 1989

A. 1.0 tesla units B. 5.0 tesla units
C. 7.0 tesla units D. 10 tesla units

21. During radiotherapy, the Buccal mucosa exhibits radiation reaction before skin due to : Karnataka 1999

A. Rapid cellular turn-over in bone
B. Slow cellular turn-over in blood vessel
C. Rapid cellular turn-over in skin
D. Rapid cellular turn-over in mucosa

22. Most radiosensitive lung cancer is : PGI 1986; AI 1988

A. Adenocarcinoma
B. Squamous cell carcinoma
C. Anaplastic carcinoma
D. Giant cell carcinoma

23. Radiation protection shields are made up of : AIIMS 1982

A. Copper B. Silver
C. Lead D. Tin

24. Commonly used type of radiation in radiotherapy is : AIIMS 1983

A. Alpha rays B. Beta rays
C. Gamma rays D. X-rays

25. The optimum distance used in radiographic examination is : NIMHANS 1987

A. 90 - 100 cm B. 150 - 160 cm
C. 180 - 190 cm D. 200 - 210 cm

26. In ultrasonography a high frequency transducer is used : AIIMS 1986

A. To see deeper structures
B. For better resolution
C. To penetrate air
D. None of the above

27. Most commonly used mode of transmission in abdominal ultrasonography is : AIIMS 1985

A. Amplitude mode (A - mode)
B. Brightness mode (B - mode)
C. Movement mode (M - mode)
D. Doppler method

28. Out of the following phases of iodinated contrast medium enhancement, CT scan makes use of : AP 1990

A. Vascular enhancement
B. Tissue opacification
C. Opacification of urinary tract
D. Any of the above

29. CT scan picture is ideal for radiotherapy planning because : TN 1989

A. Picture is available in a T.V. monitor
B. Picture is available in a film
C. The cross-sectional picture is available
D. Any of the above

30. Filters are used to reduce : AIIMS 1984

A. Processing time
B. Amount of radiation to patient
C. Exposure time
D. None of the above

31. A liver scan of a patient with advanced cirrhosis may show large cold areas due to : AIIMS 1982

A. Hepatoma
B. Fatty replacement
C. Fibrous replacement
D. Portal systemic vascular shunting
E. All are true

32. Salivary gland scanning with 99m technetium pertechnetate will give 'hot' areas in : PGI 1982

A. Warthin's tumour B. Sjogren's syndrome
C. Carcinoma D. Mixed salivary lumour

33. Compared with direct fluoroscopy an image intensifier does all except : PGI 1981

A. Allows the perception of better details
B. Increases image brightness
C. Decreases patient radiation dose
D. Allows light during screening examination
E. Increases X-ray tube loading

34. Causes of fog in X-ray plates may be all except : PGI 1983

A. Prolonged development
B. Incomplete fixing
C. Unsafe lights
D. Films stored in hot and humid atmosphere
E. Excessive light reaching the dark room

35. Acoustic shadow in ultrasound means : AI 1994

A. Reflection of sound waves
B. Absorption of sound waves
C. Reflection of X-rays
D. All of the above

36. In the thyrotoxicosis scanning, the isotope used is : PGI 1982

A. I^{131} B. I^{132}
C. Tele cobalt D. Tc

Ans.									
17. C	18. B	19. B	20. A	21. C	22. B	23. C	24. C	25. A	26. B
27. B	28. D	29. C	30. B	31. C	32. A	33. E	34. B	35. A	36. A

37. Half life of Xenon is : AIIMS 1983
A. 2-3 days B. 3-8 days
C. 5-3 days D. 8 days

38. Dye used for myelography is : PGI 1983; Delhi 1987; AI 1994
A. Conary 320 B. Myodil
C. Dianosil D. Iopanoic acid

39. Most sensitive test for metastatic deposit is : AIIMS 1985; PGI 1989
A. Isotope scan B. CT scan
C. Skeletal scurvey D. Epilepsy
E. Vascular lesions

40. Best investigation in acute cholecystitis is : AIIMS 1985
A. Technetium scan B. HIDA scan
C. Pipida scan D. Plain X- ay abdomen

41. X-ray machine is kept at a distance of 6 feet from the photographic plate to : AIIMS 1986 ; TN 1987, 89
A. Magnify the image B. Prevent magnifications
C. Enhance contrast D. None

42. Hot nodule is seen in : PGI 1981, 88
A. Adenolymphoma B. Mixed parotid
C. Adenocystic disease D. All of the above

43. The amount of I^{131} used for a thyroid scan is : AIIMS 1985, 86
A. 5 milli curies B. 5 micro curies
C. 50 milli curies D. 50 micro curies
E. 500 milli curies

44. Drug used for Ca oesophagus is : AIIMS 1997
A. Cisplatin B. Adriamycin
C. Cyclosporin D. Actinomycin-D

45. Paramagnetic contrast dye used in NMR imaging is : AIIMS 1988
A. Technetium B. Gadolinium
C. Conary D. Gallium

46. Contra-indication for the use of NMR imaging is : AIIMS 1988
A. Psychotic patients
B. Patients on lithium
C. Intracranial metallic aneurysm clips
D. Patients receiving radiotherapy

47. Microwaves cause : AI 1988
A. Retinal detachment
B. Heating-up of tissues
C. Microscopic hemorrhages
D. Convulsions

48. Not used for brachytherapy : AIIMS 1998; AI 1999
A. Cobalt 60 B. Cesium 137
C. Iridium 192 D. Gold 198

49. In ultrasound machines, the piezo electric crystal is made of : TN 1989
A. Silicon
B. Tungsten
C. Lead stannous zirconate
D. Molybdenum

50. The mean glandular dose of radiation given to a patient on Film screen mammography and xeromammography are respectively (in rad per film) are : DNB 1990
A. 0.1 - 0.2 and 0.2 - 0.4
B. 0.2 - 0.4 and 0.1 - 0.4
C. 0.4 - 0.6 and 0.4 - 0.6
D. 0.6 - 1.0 and 0.2 - 0.4

51. In pancreatic scanning, isotope used most commonly is : Rohtak 1987
A. Chromium - 51 B. Selenium - 75
C. Technetium - 99m D. Iodine - 131

52. A secondary type of radiation is that which : AIIMS 1982
A. Scaters on contact with the patient
B. Emerges from the tube and reaches the patient
C. Emerges from the patient and reaches the film
D. Controls image distortion

53. Increased radiolucency on X-ray film denotes : AIIMS 1986
A. Greater penetrability and darker shadow
B. Decreased penetrability and whiter shadow
C. Intermediate gray density
D. Same as increased density

54. X-ray attenuation depends on : AIIMS 1985
A. Bone density and molecular weight
B. Tissue density
C. Absorption coefficient
D. Tissue density and atomic number

55. Diagnostic ultrasonography is based on : DNB 1991
A. Slit beam B. Single X-ray source
C. Pulse-echo principle D. None of the above

56. Least resolution is observed in : Rajasthan 1993; Orissa 1994
A. Conventional X-ray B. Ultrasonography
C. CT Scan D. MRI Scan

57. Poor screen contact reduces : AIIMS 1981
A. Distortion B. Definition
C. Contrast D. Density

58. To decrease magnification use : AIIMS 1983
A. Increased grid ratio
B. Increased focal spot size
C. Shorter focal film distance
D. Increased target film distance

Ans.									
37. C	38. B	39. A	40. B	41. B	42. A	43. B	44. A	45. B	46. C
47. B	48. A	49. C	50. A	51. B	52. A	53. A	54. C	55. C	56. A
57. B	58. D								

59. **In radiographic quality, one of the greatest problems is considered to be : AMC 1984**
A. Technician B. Fog
C. Equipment D. Patient

60. **In radiographic quality, densities are directly controlled by : AIIMS 1983**
A. Age of patient
B. Screen contact
C. Object film distance
D. Milliampere seconds and target film distance

61. **In radiographic quality, contrast is directly controlled by : AIIMS 1983**
A. Time B. Kilovolt peak
C. Target film distance D. Milliampere

62. **A criteria for attaining satisfactoy radiographic quality would be : AIIMS 1984**
A. Always use compression
B. Target film distance and object film distance are equal
C. Part examined should be fully penetrated
D. Proper selection of patient size

63. **The use of secretin may be useful in : AMC 1984**
A. Hepatic arteriography
B. Pancreatic angiography
C. Portography
D. Superior mesenteric arteriography

64. **Spot out the wrong statement about a real time ultrasound system : AIIMS 1981**
A. Sometimes contains a moving acoustic mirror.
B. Is of particular value is obstetrics.
C. Sometimes contains transducer elements oriented with their transmitting surfaces forming the circumference of a circle.
D. Is used to measure blood flow velocity.

65. **Concentration of barium salt is very important in double Contrast Barium Meal examination, it should be : AIIMS 1985**
A. 95% w/v B. 75% w/v
C. 50% w/v D. 25% w/v

66. **Which of the following elements has got maximum half-value layer thickness (H.V.L) AI 1988**
A. Cellophone B. Aluminium
C. Copper D. Lead

67. **One Gray is equivalent to —— Rads : Rajasthan 1993**
A. 10 B. 100
C. 2000 D. 10000

68. **Colour brain scanning is done by using : AIIMS 1983**
A. Conary B. Mercury
C. Technetium D. Phosphorus

69. **In Positron Emission Tomography (PET) the following positron emitting radionuclides may be used except : AIIMS 1987**
A. O2
B. CO2
C. 18 FDG (18F2-deoxyglucose)
D. None of the above

70. **Administration of above radionuclides give information regarding : AIIMS 1987**
A. Oxygen uptake B. Blood flow
C. Glucose utilization D. All of the above

71. **For regional cerebral blood flow (CBF) studies, use inhalations or injection of : Rohtak 1989**
A. O_2 B. CO_2
C. Xenon D. Ether

72. **In MRI, images of body part are produced due to : AIIMS 1993**
A. H+ B. CO2
C. O2 D. N2

73. **Isotop renogram is : Karnataka 1994**
A. Study of renin mechanism.
B. Contrast study of kidneys, ureter and bladder.
C. Utilized in mapping the anatomy of kidneys.
D. Graphic representation of radioactivity of kidneys.

74. **Hot spot on Tm Scan in parotid is seen in : PGI 1994**
A. Adenolymphoma B. Mixed parotid tumour
C. Calculus D. Mumps

75. **Radio pharmacologic agent used for estimating GFR is : Delhi 1993; AI 1995, 99**
A. 99Tc DMSA B. 99Tc DTPA
C. 99Tc MAG D. 99Tc GHA

76. **Best imaging modality to diagnose liver mass is : AP 1993**
A. Plain film B. Angiography
C. C.T. Scan D. Nuclear scan

77. **NMR spectroscopy is based on : Rajasthan 1989, 90**
A. Diffraction B. Emission
C. Absorption D. Radiation

78. **Maximum radiation exposure is caused by : Rajasthan 1993; MP 1993**
A. Sonography B. CT Scan
C. Chest X-ray D. MRI

79. **Longest wave length is : Rajasthan 1992, 93**
A. OC waves B. Gamma waves
C. Beta waves D. X-rays

80. **Ultrasound wavelength is —— MHZ : TN 1989; Rajasthan 1992; PGI 1995, 96**
A. Below 1 B. 1-10
C. 10-20 D. Above 20

Ans.										
	59. B	60. D	61. B	62. C	63. B	64. D	65. A	66. D	67. B	68. C
	69. D	70. D	71. C	72. A	73. D	74. A	75. B	76. D	77. C	78. B
	79. A	80. D								

81. Ion which scatters X-ray more is : AI 1996
A. H+ B. Ca++
C. Lead D. Hg

82. Part of cell cycle most sensitive to radiotherapy is : AI 1996
A. S B. M
C. G_2M D. G-Phase

83. Atomic weight is : Delhi 1996
A. Protons only B. Neutrons only
C. a + b D. Electrons only

84. DOC in molor pregnancy is : JIPMER 1997
A. Actinomycin-D B. Bleomycin
C. Methotrexate D. Cyclophosphamide

85. In Ionizing radiotherapy : AI 1997
A. Pyrimidine diamers used
B. Linear entery transfers
C. Orbital electrons are affected
D. All of the above

86. Maximum penetration amongst laser is of : Rajasthan 1994
A. Xenon B. Argon
C. YAG D. CO2

87. 'Target angle' in Tele-therapy X-ray tube is : Rajasthan 1994
A. 17 B. 45
C. 30 D. 60

88. P 32 has half life of 14 days. The activity of 10 m curie dose after 42 days remains : Rajasthan 1995
A. 4 cm curie B. 1.25 m curie
C. 0.5 m curie D. None

89. True about radio isotope scanning of spleen is : Rajasthan 1996
A. Tumours & cysts can be differentiated
B. Tumours & cysts can not be differentiated
C. Not useful
D. Not indicated

90. In Teletherapy Electromagnetic wave or particulate Radiation is kept at a distance of : Karnataka 1995
A. 150 cm B. 100 cm
C. 75 cm D. 200 cm

91. Radiation is not used in : U.P. 1996
A. CAT scan
B. NMR
C. Digital substraction imaging
D. Thyroid scan

92. Half life of Au198 is——— days : DNB 1996
A. 1.3 B. 2.7
C. 3.7 D. 7.1

93. Brachy and tele therapy, both can be given by : PGI 1997
A. Ir B. Se
C. Chr D. Co

94. Benign condition treated by Radiotherapy is : AIIMS 1997
A. Pituitary adenoma B. T.B.
C. Sarcoidosis D. Melanoma

95. Least sensitive to radiation is : AIIMS 1997; IAM 2000
A. Gonads B. Kidney
C. Cartilage D. Bladder

96. Radiosensitising substance include : AIIMS 1997
A. BUDR B. Cyclophosphamide
C. 5-FU D. Hydroxyurea

97. The following tumours respond very well to irradiation therapy except : TNPSC 1997
A. Squamous cell carcinoma
B. Seminoma
C. Brain tumour
D. Soft tissue sarcoma

98. Radiation hazard is calculated in : JIPMER 1997
A. REM B. Curie
C. Rad D. Bequerol

99. Brachytherapy with radium is not used now-a-days because of : JIPMER 1998
A. Short half life
B. Need for frequent replacement
C. Generation of radon gas
D. All of the above

100. Earliest manifestation of radiation toxicity is : JIPMER 1998
A. Erythema B. Pigmentation
C. Edema D. Vesication

101. The drug of choice for chemotherapy of retinoblastoma is : MP 1998
A. 5 FU B. Hydroxyurea
C. Vincristine D. Nitrogen mustard

102. Most radiosensitive cancer among the following is : JIPMER 1998; AI 2001
A. Basal cell Ca skin
B. Squamous cell Ca Cx
C. Small cell Ca lung
D. Hepatocellular carcinoma

103. Which of the following is anti-metabolite : JIPMER 1992
A. Nitrogen mustard B. Procarbazine
C. 5 Fluoro uracil D. Cyclophosphamide

104. Poor wound healing is seen with : AIIMS 1992
A. Nitrogen mustard B. 5 flurouracil
C. Adriamycin D. Methotrexate

105. Radiation during childhood can cause : AIIMS 1992
A. Lymphoma B. Papillary Ca. Thyroid
C. Ca stomach D. Laryngeal Ca.

Ans.									
81. B	82. C	83. C	84. C	85. D	86. B	87. C	88. B	89. A	90. B
91. B	92. B	93. D	94. A	95. C	96. B	97. D	98. C	99. B	100. A
101. A	102. B	103. C	104. A	105. B					

106. Chemotherapeutic agent used in Wilim's tumor is : PGI 1993
A. Methotrexate B. Cyclophosphamide
C. 5FU D. Actinomycin-D

107. Leukoencephalopathy is seen with the use of : PGI 1993
A. Vincristine B. Cyclophosphamide
C. Methotrexate D. 5 FU

108. Of the following radiations, which is not mutagenic : PGI 1993
A. Ultrasonic B. X-ray
C. U-V rays D. Beta rays

109. X-rays are generated from : JIPMER 1993
A. Electrons B. Protons
C. Neutrons D. Electromagnetic waves

110. Lymphocytes are damaged with a radiation dosage of : JIPMER 1993
A. 5 rads B. 10 rads
C. 20 rads D. 100 rads

111. The half life of I^{131} is : TN 1993
A. 8 hours B. 2 days
C. 8 days D. 12 days

112. Which is not associated with radiation hazard : AI 1993
A. X-ray B. CAT scan
C. MRI D. PET

113. T 1/2 of Tritium is : AI 1993
A. 6 days B. 12 days
C. 6 years D. 12 years

114. In which condition the Radioisotope is not taken up : AI 1993
A. Pseudoarthrosis B. Acute osteomyelitis
C. Osteosarcoma D. Acute fracture

115. Cobalt 60 is : Delhi 1993
A. Naturally occurring radioisotope
B. Artificial radioisotope
C. A + B
D. Generates from synthesis of uranium

116. Curie is the unit for : Delhi 1993
A. Radiation emitted B. Radiation absorbed
C. Radioactivity D. All of the above

117. Radiation pneumonitis following therapy may be distinguished in part, from other pathologic condition by : PGI 1983
A. Location
B. Presence of cavitation
C. Presence of pleural fluid
D. Lack of nodularity

118. Substance which offers preferential radio-protection to tissues is/are : AIIMS 1982
A. Cysteine
B. Thiophosphate WR 2721
C. Metronidazole
D. A and B are correct
E. Only C is correct

119. One of the following radio isotopes is used for interstitial therapy : Orissa 1999
A. Phosphorus 32 B. Iodine 131
C. Indium 191 D. Gold 198

120. Isotope that concentrates selectively in abscess cavity is : TN 1993
A. Gallium B. Technetium
C. Selentum D. Chromium

121. $99Tc^{m}$ HIDA shows the normal gall bladder and biliary tract in ——— min. DNB 1994
A. 15 B. 30
C. 60 D. 120

122. Deleterious effect of ultrasound on small organisms is : DNB 1989
A. Ionisation B. Vacuolation
C. Cavitation D. Disintegration

123. Parathyroid gland can be assessed by : AIIMS 1984
A. Thallium scan
B. Technetium scan
C. Gallium scan
D. Plain X-ray neck
E. Thallium Technetium Substraction

124. The use of glucagon is contraindicated in : PGI 1981
A. Hypertension
B. Benign prostatic hypertrophy
C. Patients taking digitalis
D. Closed angle glaucoma
E. Phaechromocytoma

125. Use of a cone results in films of : AMU 1986
A. Higher contrast B. Low contrast
C. Less motion D. Long scale contrast

W126. When bones show a 'Bone-within-bone' appearance, this is indicative of : PGI 1982
A. Sickle cell anaemia
B. Bone infarction
C. Osteopetrosis
D. Chronic myelogenous leukaemia

127. X-ray films are least sensitive to which coloured light : PGI 1983
A. Violet B. Blue
C. Yellow D. Red

128. The photosensitive material used in X-rays films consists of : AIIMS 1986
A. Cellulose B. Silver bromide
C. Zine sulphide D. Cadmium tungstate

Ans. 106. D 107. A 108. A 109. D 110. D 111. C 112. C 113. D 114. A 115. B
116. C 117. A 118. D 119. D 120. A 121. B 122. C 123. E 124. E 125. A
126. A,C 127. A 128. D

129. When a X-ray film enclosed in a cassette is exposed to X-rays, the resultant exposure is by : AIIMS 1985
A. X-rays
B. Fluorescent light
C. Both by X-rays and fluorescent light
D. Neither by X-rays nor by fluorescent light

130. "Target Material" which produces X-ray in a diagnostic X-rays tube is made-up of : PGI 1983
A. Lead B Tungston
C. Cobalt D. Copper

131. The Photoelectric interaction occurs primarily in : AMU 1986
A. 'L' cell B. 'K' cell
C. Outer cell D. All shells equally

132. Radio-active iodine isotope investigation is not used in : AIIMS 1984
A. Thyroglossal fistula B. Single thyroid nodule
C. Lingula thyroid D. Carcinoma thyroid

133. Scintiphotos are best used for : AIIMS 1981
A. Radioiostope distribution data
B. Quantitative regional data
C. Both
D. None

134. The following tumors of skin are radiosensitive, except : AMU 1985
A. Cutaneous lymphoma
B. Basal cell carcinoma
C. Malignant melanoma
D. Squamous cell carcinoma

135. Radioactive phosphorus emits : AIIMS 1988
A. Only beta rays
B. X-rays
C. Only gamma rays
D. Both Beta and Gamma rays

136. Dose of radioactive phosphorus to induce a remission in polycythaemia is : AMU 1988
A. 70 micro curies B. 700 micro curies
C. 7 milli curies D. 73 milli curies

137. Outer case of radium needle is made-up of : AMC 1984
A. Plastic
B. Chromium steel
C. Platinum-irridation alloy
D. Copper-Tin alloy

138. A single whole body dose of how many rads could result in death : Rohtak 1985
A. 100 rads B. 200 rads
C. 300 rads D. 500 rads

139. Latest source of neutrons for radiotherapy is : Rohtak 1988
A. Strontium-90 B. Iodine-131
C. Californium - 252 D. Radium - 226

140. Which radiations are detected to produce a visual image in thermography : DNB 1989
A. Radio-waves B. Ultraviolet radiations
C. Infra-red radiations D. Gamma radiations

141. Gamma radiation is protected by : PGI 1987
A. Lead B. Gold
C. Copper D. Aluminium

142. Non-ionising radiation includes : AMU 1986
A. X-rays B. Beta rays
C. Gamma rays D. Infrared rays

143. Radio-active iodine uptake by thyroid is increased in : AMC 1986
A. Myxoedema B. Critinism
C. Thyrotoxicosis D. Hypoparathyroidism

144. UV rays cause : PGI 1988
A. Deletion of pyrimidines
B. Substitution of purine for pyrimidine
C. Cross-linking of purine with pyrimidine
D. Dimerisation of pyrimidine

145. Commonest post-irradiation carcinoma of thyroid is : AMU 1987
A. Papillary B. Follicular
C. Medullary D. Anaplastic

146. The biological effect of ionizing radiation is related to all except : AMU 1987
A. Dose B. Ambient pressure
C. Type of radiation D. Age of patient

147. For the side effects of radiotherapy, the factor which is not important is : AMC 1983, 87; PGI 1981
A. Type of tumour
B. Site of tumour
C. Size of tumour
D. Dose and frequency of radiation

148. Treatment by radiotherapy is most frequently indicated in carcinoma of : DNB 1989
A. Ovary B. Lung
C. Cervix D. Thyroid

149. The drug of choice for chemotherapy of retinoblastoma is : PGI 1986
A. Vincristine
B. Nitrogen mustard
C. 5-fluorouracil (5FU)
D. Triethylene melamine (TEM)

150. Ototoxicity and nephrotoxicity are frequently encountered following therapy with : UPSC 1989
A. 5-F.U B. Endoxan
C. Bleomycin D. Cis-Plantinum

151. 5-Fluoro-uracil is used in treatment of following cancers except : AIIMS 1989
A. Breast B. Stomach
C. Liver D. Mycosis fungoides

Ans.										
	129. B	130. C	131. B	132. A	133. C	134. C	135. A	136. C	137. C	138. D
	139. C	140. C	141. A	142. D	143. C	144. D	145. A	146. B	147. C	148. C
	149. A	150. D	151. D							

152. The administration of I^{131} to a thyrocardiac patient can cause all of the following except : PGI 1985
A. Carcinoma
B. Myxoedema
C. Hypoparathyroidism
D. Increase in the size of the gland

153. Permanent sterility in young woman requires radiation dosage in the range of : DNB 1991
A. 100-300 rads, single exposure
B. 300-400 rads, single exposure
C. 400-800 rads, single exposure
D. 800-1200 rads, single exposure
E. Lethal body radiation dose

154. Isotopes have same : Delhi 1987, 88
A. Number B. Weight
C. A or B D. Density

155. Anti-tumour effect of cyclophosphamide is enhanced by vitamin : NIMHANS 1988
A. A B. B2
C. B6 D. E

156. Nuclear medicine is the term used for : AIIMS 1984, 86
A. Treatment due to radiation
B. Using Radionucleotides techniques for diagnosis
C. Nucleic acid analysis
D. X-rays

157. Colon necrosis occurs at : Rajasthan 1990
A. 1000 rads B. 1500 rads
C. 2000 rads D. 2500 rads

158. Which Radio isotope is capable of displacing calcium from the body : PGI 1988
A. Radium B. Strontium
C. Plutonium D. Iridium

159. Nucleus of an atom contains : PGI 1989
A. Electrons B. Protons
C. Positrons D. Neutrons

160. Optical activity of organic substances is measured by : AI 1990
A. Spectrometer B. Polarimeter
C. Photometer D. Multimeter

161. SI unit of absorbed dose of radiation is : AIIMS 1985
A. Rads B. Roentgen
C. Gray D. Curie

162. In seminoma treated with radiotherapy, 5-years survival ratio is —— %. Rajasthan 1989
A. 10 B. 20
C. 50 D. 90

163. Half life of bromide in blood is approximate : Rajasthan 1989
A. 20 min B. 2-4 hours
C. 12 days D. 3 months

164. Out of the following which is not a radio-therapy equipment : AIIMS 1983, 85
A. Betatron
B. Telecurie-cobalt 60 unit
C. Linear accelerator
D. Thimble chamber

165. Wilhelm Conard Roentgen discovered X-rays in : Delhi 1985
A. 1852 B. 1875
C. 1891 D. 1895
E. 1905

166. The weekly dose of P32 should be in the order of —— in treatment of chronic myelogenous leukaemia or chronic lymphocytic leukaemia : AIIMS 1984
A. 1 millicurie B. 10 millicurie
C. 15 millicurie D. 100 millicurie

167. The source of gamma radiation does not include : AP 1993
A. Radon seeds
B. Cobalt 60
C. Vander Graaf generator
D. Caesaium 137

168. Indicate the conditions for radioiodin therapy in hyperthyroidism : UPSC 1982
A. Hyperthyroidism with malignant exophthalmos.
B. Long preoperative preparation.
C. Previous thyroidectomy for hyper-thyroidism.
D. All of the above.

169. Radiation is most often the treatment of choice in : AIIMS 1984
A. Cancer of cervix B. Cancer of lung
C. Cancer of thyroid D. Meningiosarcoma

170. Testicular tumour which responds best to radiation is : Delhi 1986; UPSC 1986
A. Teratoma
B. Seminoma
C. Embryonal cell carcinoma
D. None of the above

171. The utility of adjuvant radiotherapy in the treatment of tumours is limited by all the following considerations except : AP 1992
A. Injury to normal tissues
B. Oncogenic potential of treatment
C. Activation of T-lymphocytes
D. Systemic subclinical disease

172. Radiotherapy is curable in : PGI 1982
A. Ewing's tumour
B. Osteosarcoma
C. Rhabdomyosarcoma
D. Squamous cell carcinoma of mouth

Ans.									
152. C	153. B	154. A	155. A	156. B	157. D	158. B	159. B	160. B	161. C
162. D	163. C	164. D	165. D	166. A	167. A	168. D	169. A	170. B	171. C
172. A									

173. Post-operative radiation is more useful in: **AIIMS 1990**

A. Adenocarcinoma of stomach
B. Squamous cell carcinoma of oral cavity
C. Wilm's tumour
D. Sarcoma of smooth muscles

174. Which of the following are radioactive : **PGI 1983, 86**

A. Co 59 B. Co60
C. I130 D. Yt 90

175. Half life of which of the following is maximum : **AMU 1985**

A. Radon B. Gallium
C. Iridium D. Tantalum

176. Radio-active gold is used in : **AIIMS 1983**

A. Bladder tumours B. Malignant ascites
C. Gliomas D. None of the above

177. Radioactive substance used for intracavity irradiation in carcinoma cervix is : **AIIMS 1980**

A. Cobalt-60 B. Cesium
C. Irridium D. I^{131}
E. Strontium

178. In a radio-active radium needles, radium chloride is mixed with some inactive chemical, now-a-days, the salt used is : **AIIMS 1982**

A. Lead sulphide B. Lead oxide
C. Barium sulphate D. Aqua regia

179. Maximum permissible dose for a year is : **UPSC 1984**

A. 1 rad B. 5 rads
C. 50 rads D. 500 rads

180. Principle used in Radiotherapy is : **AIIMS 1994**

A. Ionizing molecules B. Charring nucleoprotein
C. Infrared rays D. Ultrasonic effect

181. Radiation mainly causes cataract of —— type : **PGI 1994**

A. Anterior subcapsular B. Posterior Subcapsular
C. Nuclear D. Polar

182. Tissue most sensitive to radiation is : **AIIMS 1995**

A. Skin B. Gonads
C. Spleen D. Liver

183. Chronic radiation injury to the intestinal tract presents with all except : **Delhi 1980**

A. Malabsorption B. Mucosal atrophy
C. Intestinal perforation D. Intestinal obstruction

184. Rotating anode X-ray tubes were introduced into diagnostic radiology in order to : **AIIMS 1984**

A. Reduce patient dose
B. Distribute heart over a larger anode area
C. Allow low K.V. technique
D. Trigger the Bucky apparatus

185. Radiation can lead to the following except : **Delhi 1995**

A. Sq. Cell Carcinoma of lung
B. Liver Carcinoma
C. Thyroid Carcinoma
D. Ovarian Carcinoma

186. Law of Bergonie and Tribondeau states that the sensitivity of cells to irradiation is : **AIIMS 1982**

A. In direct proportion to degree of differentiation.
B. In direct proportion to their reproductive activity.
C. Inversely proportional to degree of differentiation.
D. Directly proportional to their reproductive activity.

187. Ionizing drug used therapeutically is : **Delhi 1996**

A. Gold B. Lead
C. Aluminium D. Magnesium

188. Real time scanner has the following advantage : **PGI 1995**

A. Cheap B. Easy to handle
C. Can be applied to AF D. Easily available

189. Which is used in Immunofluorescent studies : **PGI 1995**

A. Fluorescein isothiocyanate
B. CO2
C. CO
D. N2O

190. Investigation by radioactive uptake is diagnostic in : **PGI 1995, 97**

A. Grave's disease
B. Autonomous toxic nodule of thyroid
C. Hashimoto's disease
D. All of the above

191. Average Field strength of MRI is ———— Tesla. **AI 1997**

A. 0.5 B. 1.1
C. 5.0 D. 10.0

192. In X-ray film emulsion, gamma depends on following except : **Rajasthan 1996**

A. Patients characteristics
B. Exposure time
C. Strength of solution
D. Temperature of solution

193. True about secondary radiation grids is : **Rajasthan 1996**

A. X-rays pass parallel to grid
B. X-ray can be angulated
C. Bifocal grids can be used in either way
D. All of the above

194. Contrast in X-rays is depend on : **Assam 1995**

A. KV
B. mA
C. Duration of exposure
D. Distance between source and object

Ans.	173. C	174. B	175. D	176. C	177. B	178. C	179. B	180. A	181. B	182. B
	183. B	184. B	185. D	186. C,D	187. A	188. C	189. A	190. B	191. B	192. A
	193. D	194. B								

195. Only gamma rays are emitted by : JIPMER 1998
A. Cesium B. Iodine
C. Thallium D. Cobalt

196. False about MRI except : WB 1998
A. Invasive
B. Adverse biological effect
C. Better separation of lystic & solid lesions
D. Poor intrinsic contrast

197. Radio nucleide scan indicated in : WB 1998
A. Metastasis
B. Pain in prosthetic hip replacement
C. Suspected malignancy of bone without X-ray feature
D. All

198. Following are low frequency except : WB 1998
A. Infra red B. Ultra violet
C. Short wave diathermy D. Faradic stimulation

199. Consider the following statements about radioactive materials : CSE 1997
1. The half life varies from isotope but is constant for each isotope.
2. The danger of exposure exists as long as the decay process lasts.
3. Quantum of radiation emitted is dependent on the mass or the amount of the material.

Of these statements
A. 1, 2 and 3 are correct B. 1 and 2 are correct
C. 1 alone is correct D. 2 and 3 are correct

200. Which of the following malignant tumours is extremely resistant to radiation : MAHE 1994
A. Embryonal carcinoma
B. Fibrosarcoma
C. Lymphosarcoma
D. Squamous cell carcinoma

201. Which of the following is not an artificial radioisotope element : Delhi 1998
A. Co60 B. I125
C. Ra88 D. Tc 99

202. Intraoperative radiotherapy is given in : AIIMS 1998
A. Ca cervix B. Ca pancreas
C. Ca prostate D. Ca thyroid

203. Following is true of planned teletherapy except : AIIMS 1998
A. Co-60
B. Ir-192
C. Stimulators
D. Computer planning and M/M system

204. Radiotherapy is not used in : AIIMS 1998
A. Ca oesophagus B. Ca cervix
C. Ca stomach D. Brain tumour

205. Not used for brachy therapy : AIIMS 1998
A. Co60 B. Cs
C. Ra D. None

206. Mantle radiation is given in : Orissa 1998
A. Hodgkin's lymphoma B. Ca cervix
C. Ca thyroid D. Ca ovary

207. Extent of cardiotoxicity of chemotherapy and radiotherapy is best diagnosed by : AI 1999
A. Echocardiogram
B. ECG
C. Radionucleide scan
D. Endomyocardial biopsy

208. The radiation utilised for treating patients in Co-60 CS 137 machines are : Orissa 1998
A. Gamma Ray B. X-ray
C. Beta Ray D. Electrons

209. Commonest cancer treated by radiotherapy in India : Orissa 1999
A. CA Rectum B. CA Cervix
C. CA Liver D. CA Stomach

210. The patient who has dental extraction before radiotherapy needs : Karnataka 1999
A. No time for healing
B. Adequate time for healing
C. Radiotherapy is not advised
D. Wait for one day to start radiotherapy

211. When infection is present in the part of the bone which received radiotherapy : Karnataka 1999
A. Response to radiotherapy is good
B. Fast healing
C. More destruction of bone
D. Tumour regression is not affected

212. Ortho voltage range : Kerala 1999
A. 100-200 kvp B. 250-300 kvp
C. 400-600 kvp D. 600-900 kvp

213. Radiosensitization is increased by following except : Kerala 1999
A. Nitroimidazole B. Molecular O2
C. Hyperbaric O2 D. Anaemia

214. In treatment by radiation, rays used are : PGI 1999
A. $\alpha\beta\varepsilon$ B. $\alpha\varepsilon\gamma$
C. $\beta\varepsilon\gamma$ D. $\alpha\beta\gamma$

215. Which of the following is true of Californium 252: Kerala 2000
A. Produced by disintegration of Plutonium.
B. Produced by neutron bombardment of Plutonium.
C. Naturally occurring Isotope.
D. Produced by disintegration of Cobalt.
E. Not useful in intracavitary therapy.

216. Radium-226 emits : PGI 2000
A. α rays B. β rays
C. γ rays D. All of the above

Ans.									
195. A	196. C	197. D	198. B	199. A	200. A	201. C	202. B	203. B	204. C
205. A	206. A	207. D	208. A	209. B	210. B	211. C	212. B	213. D	214. D
215. B	216. C								

217. Common isotopes used in interstitial and mould therapy are the following except : Kerala 2000

A. Iridium 192 B. Cobalt 60
C. Caesium 137 D. Gold 198
E. Phosphorus 32

218. Which of the following is the correct dose in Total Body Irradiation in Bone Marrow Transplantation : Kerala 2000

A. 1000 cgy-1200 cgy B. 500 cgy - 800 cgy
C. 10,000 r D. 1150 cgy
E. None of the above

219. 5-Fluoro-uracil is used in treatment of following cancers except : AI 1988

A. Stomach B. Liver
C. Breast D. Mycosis fungoides

220. The following chemotherapeutic drugs is cardio toxic : AI 1988

A. Cycloserine B. Bleomycin
C. Nitrogen mustard D. Adriamycin

221. Ototoxicity and nephrotoxicity are frequently encountered following therapy with : AI 1989

A. Bleomycin B. Endoxan
C. Cis-Platinum D. 5.F.U.

222. Extent of cardiotoxicity of chemotherapy and radiotherapy is best diagnosed by : AI 1989

A. Echocardiogram B. ECG
C. Radionucleide scan D. Endomyocardial biopsy

223. Radio sensitizer substance is : Rajasthan 2001

A. BUDR B. Methotrexate
C. 5-FU D. Cyclophosphamide

224. Most radiosensitive sarcoma is : Kerala 2001

A. Liposarcoma B. Fibrosarcoma
C. Chondrosarcoma D. Ewings sarcoma

225. Bequeral is the unit for : Kerala 2001

A. Radiation absorbed B. Radioactivity
C. Radiation emitted D. None of the above

226. Which of the following are radioactive emissions : Kerala 2001

A. Alpha B. Beta
C. Alpha & beta D. Alpha beta & gamma

227. Radiation effectiveness is least likely to be affected by : Kerala 2001

A. Phase of cell cycle
B. Active protein synthesizing cells
C. Oxygen concentration
D. Radiosensitizers

228. In gamma camera, the emissions are best detected by : JIPMER 2002

A. Geiger Muller Counter B. Densimeter
C. Scintillation Counter D. All of the above

229. Which of the following is a naturally occurring radioactive substance in the body in small quantities : JIPMER 2002

A. Radium - 226 B. Bismuth - 60
C. Iodine - 131 D. Potassium - 40

230. A 15-years old boy received radiotherapy for epndymoma of cervical cord. He gains weight after 3 months. Most probable cause is : AIIMS 2002

A. Hypothyroidism
B. Suppression of hypothalamic axis
C. Steroid intake
D. Hypopituitarism

231. In a patient with carcinoma cervix, radiotherapy is to be given. At a point 2.5 cms from source the radiation exposure is 1000 rads. What would be the radiation exposure at a point 5 cms from the source : SGPGI 2002

A. 250 rads B. 500 rads
C. 750 rads D. 1000 rads

232. Cobalt-60 on decay gives : Maharashtra 2000

A. Cobalt - 59 B. Iron
C. Cobalt-70 D. Nickel-60

233. Half life (t1/2) of a radioactive material depends upon : A.P. 2002

A. Initial concentration
B. Disintegration constant
C. Plasma protein binding
D. Route of administration

234. Gender plays an important role in which of the following radiation associated cancer : A.P. 2002

A. Lung cancer B. Thyroid cancer
C. Bone sarcoma D. CNS tumors

235. Which of the following is the most radiosensitive phase of the cell cycle : AIIMS 2002

A. GI B. S
C. G2 D. M

236. Which of the following is the most penetration beam : AI 2004

A. Electron beam B. 8 MV photons
C. 18 MV photons D. Proton beam

237. The radiation tolerance of whole liver is: AI 2004

A. 15 Gy B. 30 Gy
C. 40 Gy D. 45 Gy

238. In which malignancy post-operative radiotherapy is minimally used: AI 2004

A. Head and Neck B. Stomach
C. Colon D. Soft tissue sarcomas

239. Gamma camera in Nuclear Medicine is used for : AI 2005

A. Organ imaging
B. Measuring the radioactivity
C. Monitoring the surface contamination
D. RIA

Ans.									
217. E	218. A	219. D	220. D	221. C	222. D	223. D	224. D	225. A	226. D
227. B	228. B	229. D	230. A	231. A	232. A	233. B	234. B	235. D	236. C
237. B	238. B	239. B							

240. The technique employed in radiotherapy to counteract the effect of tumour motion due to breathing is known as : **AI 2005**

A. Arc technique
B. Modulation
C. Gating
D. Shunting

241. At t-0 there are 6 x 1023 radioactive atoms of a substance, which decay with a disintegration constant (*) equal to 0.01/sec. What would be the initial decay rate : **AI 2005**

A. 6 x 1023
B. 6 x 1022
C. 6 x 1021
D. 6 x 1023

242. Hounsfield Units depends on : **AIIMS 2009**

A. Electron density
B. Mass density
C. Effective atomic number
D. Attenuation coefficient

243. Stereotactic surgery includes all except : **AIIMS 2009**

A. Linear accelerator
B. Proton
C. Electron
D. Gamma knife

244. Which of the following therapeutic mode is commonly used in intra-operative radiotherapy : **Delhi 2009**

A. Electron
B. Photon
C. X-ray
D. Gamma-ray

245. The technique employed in radiotherapy to counter act the effect of tumour motion due to breathing is known as : **Delhi 2009**

A. Arc technique
B. Modulation
C. Gating
D. Shunting

Ans. 240. C 241. C 242. D 243. C 244. A 245. C

EXPLANATIONS OF RADIATION PHYSICS & RADIOTHERAPY

1. Ans.— A. Lymphocyte
2. Ans.— E. Henri Bacquerol
3. Ans.— E. 5 rads
4. Ans.— E. All of the above
5. Ans.— C. Has a low density
6. Ans.— D. Gamma rays
7. Ans.— C. Infrared radiation
8. Ans.— D. Thermoluminescence dose meter
9. Ans.— B. Iodine - 131
10. Ans.— B. 30 deg
11. Ans.— A. Acute lymphatic leukaemia after remission
12. Ans.— A. Carcinoma Cervix
13. Ans.— B. Bone marrow

    Lymphocyte is most radiosensitive.
14. Ans.— A. Nervous tissue
15. Ans.— C. Emerges from the tube and reaches the patient.
16. Ans.— A. Reducing scattered radiation
17. Ans.— C. 120 - 150 Kvp
18. Ans.— B. Piezoelectric
19. Ans.— B. Proton
20. Ans.— A. 1.0 tesla units
21. Ans.— C. Rapid cellular turn-over in skin
22. Ans.— B. Squamous cell carcinoma

    Anaplastic, small cell, lung tumor responds best to radiotherapy. Radiotherapy is useful in irremovable tumors or to relieve up vena caval or bronchial obstruction or involvement of spine.
23. Ans.— C. Lead
24. Ans.— C. Gamma rays
25. Ans.— A. 90 - 100 cm
26. Ans.— B. For better resolution
27. Ans.— B. Brightness mode (B - mode)
28. Ans.— D. Any of the above
29. Ans.— C. The cross-sectional picture is available
30. Ans.— B. Amount of radiation to patient
31. Ans.— C. Fibrous replacement
32. Ans.— A. Warthin's tumour

    Sialography is performed by injecting either the parotid or submaxillary duct, 1-2 ml of viscous or water soluble contrast medium.
33. Ans.— E. Increases X-ray tube loading
34. Ans.— B. Incomplete fixing
35. Ans.— A. Reflection of sound waves
36. Ans.— A. I^{131}
37. Ans.— C. 3-5 days
38. Ans.— B. Myodil

    Myodil is preferred in myelography. Urografin is used in angiography. Conray 120 in IVP.
39. Ans.— A. Isotope scan
40. Ans.— B. HIDA scan
41. Ans.— B. Prevent magnifications
42. Ans.— A. Adenolymphoma

    It takes-up radioactive iodine.
43. Ans.— B. 5 micro curies
44. Ans.— A. Cisplatin
45. Ans.— B. Gadolinium
46. Ans.— C. Intracranial metallic aneurysm clips

    Pacemakers and replacement heart valves are also contraindications.
47. Ans.— B. Heating-up of tissues
48. Ans.— A. Cobalt 60
49. Ans.— C. Lead stannous zirconate
50. Ans.— A. 0.1 - 0.2 and 0.2 - 0.4
51. Ans.— B. Selenium - 75

    This is most useful in pancreatic cancer.
52. Ans.— A. Scaters on contact with the patient
53. Ans.— A. Greater penetrability and darker shadow.

54. **Ans.— C. Absorption coefficient**

55. **Ans.— C. Pulse-echo principle**

56. **Ans.— A. Conventional X-ray**

57. **Ans.— B. Definition**

58. **Ans.— D. Increased target film distance**

59. **Ans.— B. Fog**

60. **Ans.— D. Milliampere seconds and target film distance.**

61. **Ans.— B. Kilovolt peak**

62. **Ans.— C. Part examined should be fully penetrated.**

63. **Ans.— B. Pancreatic angiography**

64. **Ans.— D. Is used to measure blood flow velocity.**

65. **Ans.— A. 95% w/v**

66. **Ans.— D. Lead**

It is also used to protect from radiation.

67. **Ans.— B. 100**

68. **Ans.— C. Technetium**

69. **Ans.— D. None of the above**

70. **Ans.— D. All of the above**

71. **Ans.— C. Xenon**

72. **Ans.— A. H+**

73. **Ans.— D. Graphic representation of radioactivity of kidneys.**

In addition to the large and costly magnet required for MRI, the machine also uses pulses of radiowaves.

74. **Ans.— A. Adenolymphoma**

75. **Ans.— B. 99Tc DTPA**

DTPA is used to assess perfusion, GFR, obstructive uropathy and vesicoureteric reflux. DMSA is used for cortical masses.

76. **Ans.— D. Nuclear scan**

77. **Ans.— C. Absorption**

78. **Ans.— B. CT Scan**

79. **Ans.— A. OC waves**

80. **Ans.— D. Above 20**

81. **Ans.— B. Ca++**

82. **Ans.— C. G_2M**

83. **Ans.— C. a + b**

84. **Ans.— C. Methotrexate**

85. **Ans.— D. All of the above**

86. **Ans.— B. Argon**

87. **Ans.— C. 30**

88. **Ans.— B. 1.25 m curie**

89. **Ans.— A. Tumours & cysts can be differentiated**

90. **Ans.— B. 100 cm**

91. **Ans.— B. NMR**

92. **Ans.— B. 2.7**

93. **Ans.— D. Co**

94. **Ans.— A. Pituitary adenoma**

95. **Ans.— C. Cartilage**

Gonads and Bone marrow are most sensitive.

96. **Ans.— B. Cyclophosphamide**

97. **Ans.— D. Soft tissue sarcoma**

98. **Ans.— C. Rad**

99. **Ans.— B. Need for frequent replacement**

100. **Ans.— A. Erythema**

101. **Ans.— A. 5 FU**

102. **Ans.— B. Squamous cell Ca Cx**

Among the given tumors, Ca cervix is most radio-sensitive.

103. **Ans.— C. 5 Fluoro uracil**

104. **Ans.— A. Nitrogen mustard**

105. **Ans.— B. Papillary Ca. Thyroid**

106. **Ans.— D. Actinomycin-D**

107. **Ans.— A. Vincristine**

108. **Ans.— A. Ultrasonic**

109. **Ans.— D. Electromagnetic waves**

110. **Ans.— D. 100 rads**

111. **Ans.— C. 8 days**

112. **Ans.— C. MRI**

In this, magnetic field is used.

113. **Ans.— D. 12 years**

It is 12.4 years.

114. **Ans.— A. Pseudoarthrosis**

115. **Ans.— B. Artificial radioisotope**

116. **Ans.— C. Radioactivity**

117. **Ans.— A. Location**

118. **Ans.— D. A and B are correct**

119. **Ans.— D. Gold 198**

120. **Ans.— A. Gallium**

121. **Ans.— B. 30**

122. **Ans.— C. Cavitation**

123. Ans.— E. Thallium Technitium Substraction

124. Ans.— E. Phaechromocytoma

125. Ans.— A. Higher contrast

126. Ans.— A. Sickle cell anaemia and Osteopetrosis &C. Bone within bone appearance is due to endosteal new bone formation. It is seen in Normal (thoracic and lumbar vertebrae in infants and growth recovery lines after infancy), infantile cortical hyperostosis (Caffey's disease), Sickle cell disease/thalassemia, congenital syphilis, Osteopetrosis/Oxalosis, radiation, acromegaly, and Paget's disease.

127. Ans.— A. Violet

128. Ans.— D. Cadmium tungstate

129. Ans.— B. Fluorescent light

130. Ans.— C. Cobalt

131. Ans.— B. 'K' cell

132. Ans.— A. Thyroglossal fistula

133. Ans.— C. Both

134. Ans.— C. Malignant melanoma

135. Ans.— A. Only beta rays

136. Ans.— C. 7 milli curies

137. Ans.— C. Platinum-irridation alloy

138. Ans.— D. 500 rads

139. Ans.— C. Californium - 252

140. Ans.— C. Infra-red radiations

141. Ans.— A. Lead

142. Ans.— D. Infrared rays

Others are ionizing radiations.

143. Ans.— C. Thyrotoxicosis

144. Ans.— D. Dimerisation of pyrimidine

145. Ans.— A. Papillary

146. Ans.— B. Ambient pressure

147. Ans.— C. Size of tumour

148. Ans.— C. Cervix

149. Ans.— A. Vincristine

150. Ans.— D. Cis-Plantinum

151. Ans.— D. Mycosis fungoides

152. Ans.— C. Hypoparathyroidism

153. Ans.— B. 300-400 rads, single exposure

154. Ans.— A. Number

Isotopes have same numbers ("Mnemonic, Topes have numbers") whereas isobars have same weight (Mnemonic "Bars have weight").

155. Ans.— A. A

156. Ans.— B. Using Radionucleotides techniques for diagnosis.

157. Ans.— D. 2500 rads

158. Ans.— B. Strontium

159. Ans.— B. Protons

160. Ans.— B. Polarimeter

161. Ans.— C. Gray

162. Ans.— D. 90

163. Ans.— C. 12 days

164. Ans.— D. Thimble chamber

165. Ans.— D. 1895

166. Ans.— A. 1 milli curie

167. Ans.— A. Radon seeds

It is protected by lead.

168. Ans.— D. All of the above

169. Ans.— A. Cancer of cervix

170. Ans.— B. Seminoma

Dysgerminoma in female is one of the most radiosensitive tumor.

171. Ans.— C. Activation of T-lymphocytes

172. Ans.— A. Ewing's tumour

173. Ans.— C. Wilm's tumour

174. Ans.— B. Co60

175. Ans.— D. Tantalum

Cobalt-60 has a half life of 5.26 years. Half life of cobalt 57 is 270 days and Cobalt 58 is 71.3 days.

176. Ans.— C. Gliomas

177. Ans.— B. Cesium

178. Ans.— C. Barium sulphate

179. Ans.— B. 5 rads

180. Ans.— A. Ionizing molecules

181. Ans.— B. Posterior Subcapsular

182. Ans.— B. Gonads

183. Ans.— B. Mucosal atrophy

184. Ans.— B. Distribute hear over a larger anode area.

185. Ans.— D. Ovarian Carcinoma

186. Ans.— C. and D. Inversely proportional to degree of differentiation and Directly proportional to their reproductive activity.

187. Ans.— A. Gold

188. Ans.— C. Can be applied to AF

189. Ans.— A. Fluroescein isothiocyanate

Half life of gold-198 is 2.7 days.

190. Ans.— B. Autonomous toxic nodule of thyroid

191. Ans.— B. 1.1

The field strengths used are 0.15 to 1.5 Tesla (1500 to 15000 Gauss).

192. Ans.— A. Patients characteristics

193. Ans.— D. All of the above

194. Ans.— B. mA

195. Ans.— A. Cesium

196. Ans.— C. Better separation of lystic & solid lesions.

197. Ans.— D. All

198. Ans.— B. Ultra violet

199. Ans.— A. 1, 2 and 3 are correct

200. Ans.— A. Embryonal carcinoma

201. Ans.— C. Ra88

202. Ans.— B. Ca pancreas

203. Ans.— B. Ir-192

204. Ans.— C. Ca stomach

Adenocarcinoma is not highly radiosensitive.

205. Ans.— A. Co60

206. Ans.— A. Hodgkin's lymphoma

207. Ans.— D. Endomyocardial biopsy

208. Ans.— A. Gamma Ray

209. Ans.— B. CA Cervix

210. Ans.— B. Adequate time for healing

211. Ans.— C. More destruction of bone

212. Ans.— B. 250-300 kvp

Lack of oxygen makes it radioresistant.

213. Ans.— D. Anaemia

214. Ans.— D. abg

215. Ans.— B. Produced by neutron bombardment of Plutonium.

216. Ans.— C. γ rays

217. Ans.— E. Phosphorus 32

218. Ans.— A. 1000 cgy-1200 cgy

219. Ans.— D. Mycosis fungoides

5-FU is also used in colorectal cancer, endocrine tumors (insulinoma and gastrinonas).

220. Ans.— D. Adriamycin

Daunorubicin (arrythmia, cardiomyopathy) and rarely bleomycin (chest pain), other cardiotoxic anticancer drugs.

221. Ans.— C. Cis-Platinum

Other ototoxic drugs are bleomycin and mustine and nephrotoxic is cyclophosphamide

222. Ans.— D. Endomyocardial biopsy

Histology helps in confirming diagnosis.

223. Ans.— D. Cyclophosphamide

224. Ans.— D. Ewings sarcoma

225. Ans.— A. Radiation absorbed

226. Ans.— D. Alpha beta & gamma

227. Ans.— B. Active protein synthesizing cells

228. Ans.— B. Densimeter

229. Ans.— D. Potassium - 40

230. Ans.— A. Hypothyroidism

231. Ans.— A. 250 rads

232. Ans.— A. Cobalt - 59

233. Ans.— B. Disintegration constant

234. Ans.— B. Thyroid cancer

235. Ans.— D. M

236. Ans.— C. 18 MV photons

237. Ans.— B. 30 Gy

The whole liver can receive 20-30 Gy, with an upper threshold of 33-35 Gy and onset of radiation hepatopathy at more than 35 Gy.

238. Ans.— B. Stomach

239. Ans.— B. Measuring the radioactivity

* Capromab pendetide is an indium-labelled intact murine IgG1 monoclonal antibody reactive with prostate specific membrane antigen expressed by prostate tissue (used as a imaging agent for the detection of metastasis).

* To achieve optical image resolution, it is crucial to obtain adequate count density while at same time minimizing motion artifact that it is likely to occur it s acquisition timer are too prolonged. For this reason, "In Capromab pendetide spect imaging should be done on multiheaded large field of view GAMMA CAMERAS. (Measures the radioactivity of "Indium-labelled monoclonal antibody".

240. Ans.— C. Gating

"Another approach to account of the effects of respiratory motion is gating in which irradiation is delivered only at specified times in the patient's respiratory cycle"

* In the deep inspiration breath hold technique patients are instructed to hold their breath at or slightly below deep inspiration.

* In active breathing control technique, patient's respiratory cycle is monitored with a spirometer. At a specified point in the cycle, a valve closes the air supply to the patient and the Linear accelerator is turned on.

241. Ans.— C. 6 x 1021

Decay rate (dN/dt) = - N

Where, N= number of radioactive nuclei

l = Decay constant

-Minus sign indicates that the number of nuclei is decreasing with time.

Now, put the values given in the question.

Decay rate = $0.01 \times 6 \times 10^{23}$

= -6×10^{21}

242. Ans.— D. Attenuation coefficient

There is a linear relationship between voxel signal intensity (image brightness) and the X-ray linear attenuation coefficient (μ), which is scaled relatively to air and water and expressed in Hounsfield units (H).

243. Ans.— C. Electron

It is a high precision, stereotactically guided delivery of larg dose of radiation in a single fraction. It can be delivered with the 'gamma knife' (Option-D) consisting of multiple cobalt-60 radioactive sources or X-rays from linear accelerator (Option A).

244. Ans.— A. Electron

245. Ans.— C. Gating

SHORT TEXTBOOK OF PSYCHIATRY
(Aids to Psychiatry)

About this Book (New Edition)

- This new book is specificially written for easy grasping of Psychiatry in a clearent, pointwise, simple and easy understandable language and is exlusively based on the ***examination oriented*** pattern.
- A list of headings important for ***Undergraduate*** and ***Postgraduate examinations*** are given at the starting
- Various ***Question Papers*** of Psychiatry from previous years of many national undergraduate examinations have been added at the end of book.
- ***Multiple Choice Questions (MCQ's)***, asked on various Undergraduate and Postgraduate Examinations have been added at the end of book
- Each chapter ends with ***important points*** enlisted in abox
- A section on the general principles of Psychiatry with a special emphasis on the Historical aspects (indian/Western), ***Symptomatology*** and Psychiatric Examination has been included.
- An updated section on Psychiatric Treatments including newer advances and list of all ***Psychotropic Drugs*** in alphabetically order (according to trade names) have been added.
- Important detailed chapters on Indian Psychiatry (Contributions of Indian Psychiatrists, Epidemiology of various disorders, National Mental Health Programme of India, Forensic Psychiatry, Indian culture bound syndromes etc).
- An important list of appendices include ***Psychiatric Glossary,*** list of ***Psychological Tests, Psychiatric Side effects of Medical Drugs*** etc.
- Useful book for various Medical Competitive and Undergraduate Examination; Civil Services Examinations
- Edited by : ***Dr. M.S. Bhatia*** (M.D., Dip. W.P.A.) an experienced teacher and examiner, associated with editing of many popular books on undergraduate and Postgraduate Examinations.

8

IMPORTANT TEXT OF RADIOIMAGING

INVESTIGATIONS

MAJOR INDICATIONS FOR ULTRASOUND EXAMINATION

I. **Chest**
- A. *Pleural fluid*
  1. Determination
  2. Thoracentesis

II. **Cardiovascular**
- A. *Aorta*
  1. Aneurysm
  2. Graft evaluation
- B. *Echocardiography*

III. **Renal**
- A. *Mass*
  1. Cyst
  2. Tumor
  3. Other (inflammatory)
  4. Follow up
- B. *Hydronephrosis detection*
- C. *Nephrolithiasis*
  1. Detection
  2. Follow up
- D. *Cystic renal disease; Adult*
- E. *Biopsy localization*
- F. *Renal transplant evaluation*

IV. **Gastrointestinal**
- A. *Liver*
  1. Mass
     - a) Neoplasm
     - b) Primary
       - i) Malignant
       - ii) Benign
     - c) Abscess
     - d) Cyst
  2. Diffuse alteration - cirrhosis
- B. *Pancreas*
  1. Mass
     - a. Solid (tumor)
     - b. Fluid (pseudocyst)
  2. Pancreas
- C. *Biliary system*
  1. Cholelithiasis
  2. Ductal dilatation - jaundice
     - a) Intrahepatic
     - b) Extrahepatic
  3. Acute or chronic cholecystitis
  4. Carcinoma of the gall bladder
  5. Adenomyosis of the gall-bladder
  6. Polyp of the gall-bladder
- D. *Spleen*
  1. Size
  2. Trauma-infarction or haemorrhage
  3. Mass
     - a) Neoplasm
     - b) Cyst

V. **Retroperitoneal**
- A. *Lymphadenopathy*

VI. **Pelvic**
- A. *Gynaecologic diseases*
  1. Uterus
     - a) Mass-benign vs malignant
     - b) IUD
     - c) Congenital anomalies
  2. Ovary
     - a) Mass-cystic disease or neoplastic disease
     - b) inflammatory - PID

3. Fallopian tubes
   a. Ectopic pregnancy
   b. Inflammatory

B. *Obstetrics*
1. Ovarian follice determination
2. Fetal progress
3. Fetal anomalies
4. Amniocentesis
5. Placenta evaluation

C. *Ascites*

D. *Pelvic adenopathy*

VII. General abdomen

A. *Ascites determination*

B. *Abdominal wall patholgoy*
1. Mass
2. Wound abscess

VIII. Genital

A. *Testicular*
1. Neoplasm
2. Infection
3. Varix
4. Torsion
5. Fluid collection

B. *Ovarian*

IX Extremity

A. *Vascular aneurysms*

B. *Mass evaluation*
1. Solid
2. Cystic

X Neonatal-premature brain imaging

MAJOR INDICATIONS FOR CT EXAMINATION

I. Head

A. *Cerebrovascular diseases*
1. Cerebral infarction
2. Intracranial haemorrhage
3. Trauma-subdural/epidural hematoma

B. *Intracranial tumors*

C. *Hydocephalus detection*

D. *Inflammatory lesions*

E. *Degenerative diseases of the CNS*
1. Brainatrophy
2. Multiple sclerosis
3. Post-operative or post-traumatic porencephaly
4. Congenital hypoplasia

II Spinal canal

A. *Herniated disc*

B. *Spinal cord tumors*

C. *Congenital anomalies*

D. *Bony abnormalities*
1. Posterior articular degenerative disease
2. Spinal stenosis

E. *Spinal trauma*

III Larynx

A. *Carcinoma*
1. Pre-operative
2. Recurrence

B. *Trauma*

IV. Chest and mediastinum

A. *Neoplasms of the lung*
1. Primary
   a. Malignant
   b. Benign
2. Metastases

B. *Mediastinal widening*
1. Vascular
2. Neoplasm
3. Lymph nodes
4. Fat

C. *Detection of occult disease*
1. Thymoma-myasthenia gravis
2. Lymph nodes

V. Cardiovascular

A. *Aortic dissection*

B. *Aortic aneurysms*

C. *Venous obstruction/thrombosis*

VI. Renal

A. *Mass*
1. Neoplasm
   a) Malignant
   b) Benign
2. Cyst
3. Inflammatory/abscess

B. *Cystic renal disease*
1. Polycystic disease; Adult

C. *Perianal extension*
1. Inflammatory
2. Haemorrhage
3. Post-transplant

VII. *Gastrointestinal*

A. *Liver*
a) Primary neoplasm
1. Malignant
2. Benign
b) Metastatic involvement
c) Abscess
d) Cyst

B. *Pancreas*
1. Mass
a) Neoplasm
1. Malignant
2. Benign
b) Pseudocyst
2. Pancreatitis
3. Biopsy guidance

C. *Spleen*
1. Trauma

VIII Adrenal

A. *Neoplasm*
1. Primary
a) Malignant
b) Benign
2. Metastatic

B. *Bilateral enlargement - Hyperplasia*

IX. Retroperitoneal

A. *Lymphadenopathy*

B. *Neoplasm*
1. Primary
2. Secondary spread

C. *Extension of inflammatory process*
1. Pancreas
2. Kidney

X. Pelvis

A. *Bladder malignancy*
1. Intrinsic
2. Perivesical extension

B. *Prostate carcinoma - extension*

C. *Pelvic lymphadenopathy*

D. *Gynaecologic tumor - extension*

E. *Bony trauma*

XI. General abdomen

A. *Tumor staging*

B. *Peritoneal mass*

XII. Musculoskeletal

A. *Tumor*
1. Malignant
2. Benign

B. *Soft tissue mass*

C. *Complex musculoskeletal anatomy*
1. Pelvis
2. Shoulder girdle
3. Sternum
4. Sternoclavicular joints
5. Accessory vertebral joints

D. *Trauma*

MAJOR INDICATIONS FOR NUCLEAR MEDICINE EXAMINATIONS

I. Central Nervous System

A. *Communicating hydrocephalus (indium-111)*

B. *Brain (rechnetium-99m-glucoheptonate)*

II. Thyroid (pertechnetate or iodine-123/131).

A. *Hyperparathyroidism*
1. Graves' disease
2. Adenoma

B. *Goiter*

C. *Thyroid mass*
1. Neoplastic disease
a) Benign
b) Malignant

D. *Metastatic detection of known thyroid carci noma (I^{131})*
1. Distant - bone
2. Local extension

E. *Therapy (I^{131})*
1. Hyperparathyroidism
2. Neoplastic suppression

III. Chest

A. *Detention of Pulmonary emboli*
1. Ventilation (Xenon-133)
2. Perfusion (technetium-99m macroaggre-gated albumin)

B. *Asymmetric perfusion of the two sides of the chest in pulmonary disease (99mTc-MAA)*

C. *Mediastinal mass - Substernal thyroid (I^{131} or pertechnetate)*

IV. Cardiovascular

A. *Ischemic heart disease: Thallium stress test (thallium-201 chloride)*

B. *Myocardial infarction detention (99Tc-pyrophosphate)*

C. *Cardiac-wall movement abnormalities and cardiac output - gated studies (99mTc-labelled RBCs)*

D. *Quantitation of right-to-left cardiac shunts (99mTc-MAA)*

V. Renal (99mTc-dimercaptosuccinic acid and I^{131} - orthoiodo hippuran)

A. Renovascular hypertension

B. Renal function

C. Transplant

D. Obstructive uropathy

VI. Gastrointestinal

A. Liver/spleen (99mTc- sulfur colloid)

1. Metastasis
2. Diffuse alterations - cirrhosis
3. Identifying ectopic splenic tissue
4. Trauma

B. *Hepatobiliary imaging (99mTc-hepatobiliary iminodiacetic acid)*

C. *Gastrointestinal bleeding*

1. Active (99m Tc-sulfur colloid)
2. Intermittent (99m Tc-labelled RBCs)

D. *Schilling test - pernicious anemia*

1. Cobalt 58 + vitamin-B12
2. Cobalt 57 + vitamin-B12

VII. General abdomen (gallium-67 citrate)

A. *Abscess*

1. Unknown location
2. Extent or response to therapy

B. *Malignancy*

1. Unknown location of primary
2. Extent/staging (e.g., lymphoma)

VIII. Genital (99m Tc-methylene dysphosphonate)

A. *Testicular torsion*

IX. Musculoskeletal (99m-Tc-methylene dysphosphonate)

A. *Bony metastasis*

B. *Osteomyelitis*

C. *Tumor extension of known bone tumor*

D. *Metabolic bone disorders*

COMPUTERIZED TOMOGRAPHY (CT)

Advantages

1. Most widely available imaging method.
2. Best understood imaging method.
3. Particularly useful for observing gross neuropathological conditions, cortical atrophy, ventricular enlargement, tumors, strokes, calcified lesions.
4. Low to Moderate cost.
5. Unsuspected specific neurological conditions may be detected.
6. Can visualise bony structures.
7. Relative simplicity.
8. Preferable for patients adversely affected by MRI e.g. pregnancy, pacemaker, aneurysmal clips etc.

Disadvantages

1. Ionizing radiation is used.
2. Limited visualizing of structure in transverse (axial) plane.
3. Poor contrast between white and grey matter.
4. Soft tissue imaging adjacent to bone poor.
5. Utility limited to focal pathology.
6. Possible allergy response to contrast media.
7. No normal controls available because of risk of radiation.

MAGNETIC RESONANCE IMAGING (MRI)

Advantages

1. Does not use ionizing radiation.
2. Visualization of structure in a variety of planes (transverse, coronal, sagittal).
3. Excellent tissue resolution particularly differentiating grey and white matter.
4. High sensitivity for detention of white matter lesions e.g. Multiple sclerosis plaques.
5. Optimal for imaging pathology of lesions.
6. Capable of imaging brain structure adjacent to bone (particularly posterior fossa structures).

7. Injection of contrast material not required.
8. Flexible imaging measurement parameters.

Disadvantages

1. More expensive and less available than CT scan.
2. Limited by conditions adversely affecting MRI magnetic field e.g. pregnancy, pacemaker, aneurysm clip, claustrophobia, ferromagnetic foreign body, calcified lesions.
3. Possibility of toxicity of ferromagnetic substance if injected as contrast media.

POSITRON EMISSION TOMOGRAPHY (PET)

Advantages

1. Capable of monitoring a broad range of biochemical processes.
2. Monitors brain metabolism and regional variations in brain activity.
3. Facilitates examination of brain neurotransmitter system particularly through receptor mapping.
4. Indicates sites of action of psychoactive drugs and can be used to monitor treatment.
5. Indicates brain activity during behaviour and cognitive functioning.
6. Good temporal resolution (less than 1 minute)
7. Good spatial resolution.
8. Sensitive to cellular dysfunction without structural pathology. So, useful in differential diagnosis of patients at risk.

Disadvantages

1. Difficult to bind especially in urban area.
2. High capital investment expenses.
3. High recurring costs.
4. Limited clinical availability.
5. Significant radiation exposure.

MAGNETIC ENCEPHALOGRAPHY (MEG)

Advantages

1. Capable of 3 dimensional localization.
2. Excellent temporal resolution.
3. Very good spatial resolution.
4. Less interference with source localization by heterogeneity of tissue structure in hand.

Disadvantages

1. Less sensitive to deep sources of activity.
2. Limited signal/noise differentiation.
3. High capital investment for instrumentation and shielded room/
4. Necessiates several long recordings.
5. Not suitable for less cooperative patients.
6. Further validation required for computer program model.
7. Many technical problems.
8. Available in very few centres.

MCQ's OF RADIOIMAGING

What is important in Radioimaging

Diagnostic views (of skull, chest, Paranasal sinuses, Effusions), Techniques (Contrast medias used esp. in Carotid angiography, Bronchography, I.V.P., Myelography etc.)

1. **Which of the following view is for styloid process : AIIMS 1981**
A. Albers-Schonberg B. Cahoon
C. Hickey D. Rhese

2. **Foetal life can be detected earlier and more consistently by : AIIMS 1982**
A. Abdominal roentgenography
B. Ultrasonic flow detector
C. Foetal ECG
D. Isotope amniography

3. **Which of the following view is for optic foramen : AIIMS 1981**
A. Water's B. Towne's
C. Valdini D. Rhese

4. **Skyline view is for : Rohtak 1986**
A. Recurrent dislocation of shoulder
B. Fracture patella
C. Fracture mandible
D. Fracture femur

5. **The congenital malformation which can be diagnosed by ultrasound at the earliest : AI 1994**
A. Hydrocephalus B. Limb aplasia
C. Anencephaly D. Renal agenesis

6. **Xeroradiography is mainly used for —— cancer : Delhi 1982**
A. Lung B. Breast
C. Thyroid D. Stomach

7. **Of the following structures, which is better visualized in a CT scan (head) in comparison to MRI (Magnetic Resonance Imaging) : PGI 1988**
A. Differentiation of Gray matter from white matter
B. Demyelinating disease
C. Differentiation of infarct and tuberculomas
D. Better visualization of bone and small calcifications

8. **In stroke, PET imaging is useful in acute studies to determine : AIIMS 1988**
A. Aetiology
B. Prognosis
C. Viable from non-viable tissue
D. All of the above

9. **MRI should be used with caution in patients with : AIIMS 1988**
A. Acute stroke B. Brain stem lesions
C. Demyelinating disease D. Cardiac pacemakers

10. **Which of the following is more like a physiological investigation : AMU 1986**
A. X-ray skull
B. CT Scan head
C. Magnetic Resonance Imaging (MRI)
D. Position Emission Tomography (PET)

11. **In demonstrating past strokes, which of the following is most sensitive : DNB 1990**
A. EEG B. CT scan
C. MRI D. Carotid angiography

12. **The definite diagnosis of cerebral lesions in AIDS is by : DNB 1992**
A. EEG B. CT scan
C. MRI D. Brain biopsy

13. **Which are the lesions in which 2-D echocardiography may not be helpful in diagnosis of : Karnataka 1989**
A. Mild mitral stenosis
B. Mild aortic incompetence
C. Pericardial effusion
D. None of the above

14. **Diagnostic investigation in retropharyngeal abscess : PGI 1993**
A. X-ray lateral view of neck in erect position.
B. X-ray lateral view of neck in extension position.
C. X-ray lateral view of neck of flexed position.
D. X-ray during inspiraion.

15. **In IVP, one can see : Delhi 1995**
A. Nephrons B. Collecting Tubules
C. Blood vessels D. None of the above

Ans.									
1. B	2. B	3. D	4. B	5. C	6. B	7. D	8. C	9. D	10. D
11. C	12. D	13. A	14. B	15. B					

16. **Gunson method of X-ray imaging is used to take images of : AP 1991**
A. Mastoid
B. PNS
C. Organic vegetable matter in the respiratory tract
D. Soft tissue image of neck

17. **Which one of the following cannot be assessed by ultrasonography : AP 1991**
A. Placental ageing
B. Foetal kidney function
C. Foetal breathing movements
D. Oesophageal atresia

18. **Sequestration lung is best diagnosed by : AP 1993**
A. C.T. Scan B. M.R.I.
C. Barium swallow D. Angiography

19. **Retroperitoneal air is not manifested by air along : AP 1993**
A. Psoas margins B. Perinephric area
C. Spleen D. Adrenals

20. **Radiolucent multiocular cyst of the body of mandible is : AP 1994**
A. Abscess B. Dental cyst
C. Dentigerous cyst D. Adamantinoma

21. **CT scanning and ultrasonography are superior to standard X-ray techniques using iodinated compounds in the evaluation of : AIIMS 1986**
A. Urinary incontinence
B. Extrinsic bladder compression
C. Urethral abnormalities
D. Cystourethral reflux
E. Intrinsic urinary tract obstruction

22. **For all sinuses, best view is : AIIMS 1982**
A. Occipito frontal B. Lateral
C. Brow up D. Mento vertical

23. **Which is not true about CT Scan : Rajasthan 1993**
A. Pancreas is the abdominal organ best suited for CT scan
B. Bone appears gray
C. Bone appears white
D. All are correct

24. **Lymphography is most commonly employed for : AIIMS 1984**
A. Tuberculosis of spine
B. Hodgkin's disease
C. Cancer kidney
D. Retroperitoneal liposarcoma

25. **Micturating cystourethrogram is not used in : AMC 1985; AI 1989**
A. Renal tumours B. Hydronephrosis
C. Urinary obstruction D. Recurrent UTI

26. **Dye used for bronchography is : Delhi 1985, 87, 88; TN 1993**
A. Iopanoic acid
B. Sodium diatrozite
C. Meglumine iodothalamte
D. Biligraffin
E. Dianosil

27. **Scintigraphy is used to demonstrate tumor in the : AMC 1985**
A. Breast B. Stomach
C. Rectum D. Vertebral column
E. Kidney

28. **Which view is used to visualize the foramina of skull : DNB 1990**
A. AP view B. Lateral view
C. Towne's view D. Base of skull view

29. **Stenver's view is used to visualize : PGI 1983**
A. Internal auditory meatus
B. Mastoid air cells
C. Optic foramina
D. Temporomandibular joint

30. **Stryker's view is used in shoulder joint to visualize : AIIMS 1985**
A. Muscle calcification
B. Recurrent subluxation
C. Sub-acromial calcification
D. Bicipital groove

31. **Adernal gland enlargement is best diagnosed by : PGI 1986**
A. Plain X-ray
B. CT scan
C. Retograde pyelography
D. IVP

32. **USS is not useful in : AI 1998**
A. CBD stones at the distal end of CBD
B. Breast cyst
C. Ascites
D. Full bladder

33. **Doppler ultrasound is used for diagnosing : AI 1998**
A. Intrauterine pregnancy
B. IUGR
C. Cardiovascular malformation
D. Neural tube defects

34. **Which of the following is fat soluble : Delhi 1993**
A. Metrizamide B. Iohexol
C. Conray 420 D. Myodil

35. **4 vessel carotid angiography is done by injecting dye into : Delhi 1993**
A. 2 ext. carotids + 2 vertebral
B. 2 int. carotids + 2 vertebral
C. 2 int. carotids + 1 vertebral
D. 2 ext. carotids + 1 vertebral

Ans.									
16. D	17. B	18. D	19. C	20. D	21. B	22. D	23. B	24. B	25. A
26. E	27. D	28. D	29. B	30. B	31. B	32. D	33. C	34. D	35. C

36. **Phlebography is done by injecting dye into :** **Delhi 1993**
A. Ant. tibial vein B. Great saphenous vein
C. Dorsal metatarsal vein D. Short saphenous vein

37. **Best investigation for vesicoureteric reflex is :** **Delhi 1993**
A. Ultrasound B. Cystoscopy
C. Micturating cystogram D. Plain X-ray abdomen

38. **The first CT scan was manufactured by :** **AIIMS 1984**
A. Hitachi, Japan
B. Mitshuhibi, Japan
C. Electromusical Instruments, England
D. General Electric, USA

39. **The substance used for OCG is :** **DNB 1989**
A. Iapanoic acid
B. Sodium diatrozite
C. Meglumine iodothalamate
D. Biligraffin
E. Dianosil

40. **Lymphography is most commonly employed for :** **Rohtak 1985**
A. Tuberculosis of spine
B. Hodgkin's disease
C. Cancer kidney
D. Retroperitoneal liposarcoma

41. **Which of the following is radiographed in the upright position to demonstrate fluid level :** **AMU 1984**
A. Sinuses B. Parotid duct
C. Mandibular menti D. Carotid artery

42. **Name the contrast medium used for intravenous cholangiography :** **PGI 1986**
A. Sodium isopaque
B. Iopanoic acid
C. Methyglucamine iodipamide
D. Methylaglucamine diatrizoate

43. **IVP is done using :** **AIIMS 1983**
A. Conary 240 B. Conary 380
C. Conary 480 D. Conary 540

44. **Percentage of cold Thyroid nodules likely to be malignant :** **AIIMS 1993**
A. 20 % B. 30 %
C. 40 % D. 72 %

45. **Double contrast barium studies were first of all used in :** **AIIMS 1986**
A. U.K. B. U.S.A.
C. Japan D. U.S.S.R.

46. **"Enteroclysis " is synonymous with :** **AIIMS 1986**
A. Hypotonic duodenography
B. Barium meal follow through
C. Small bowel enema
D. All of the above

47. **Salt of barium used in barium studies is :** **PGI 1986**
A. Barium carbonate B. Barium sulphate
C. Barium sulphide D. Barium chloride

48. **Present day indication for Bronchography is :** **AIIMS 1984, 85**
A. Bronchial cyst
B. Bronchiectasis
C. Bronchiolitis obliterans
D. Chronic bronchitis

49. **Occipitomental view is suitable for following sinuses except :** **AIIMS 1984**
A. Frontal B. Ant. Ethmoidal
C. Post. Ethmoidal D. Sphenoidal

50. **CT scan will reveal following except :** **PGI 1987**
A. Cerebral tumours
B. Cerebral haemorrhages
C. Cerebral atrophy
D. Grey and a white matter differentiation

51. **Sialography term is applied to X-ray demonstration with injection of a radiopaque media of which of the following :** **AMC 1984**
A. Lymph glands B. Axillary glands
C. Salivary glands D. Adrenal glands

52. **Seldinger needle is used for :** **UPSC 1988**
A. Selective arteriograph B. Ureterography
C. Arthrography D. Sinography

53. **The most specific non-invasive technique for diagnosis of endocrine exophthalmas is :** **PGI 1984**
A. CT scan B. MRI
C. Orbital echography D. Radionuclide scan
E. Conventional tomography

54. **On usual CT scale of densities (-1000 to +1000), brain tissue measures :** **AIIMS 1986**
A. -10 to +10 B. 0 to +20
C. +10 to +30 D. +20 to +45
E. +50 to +100

55. **Which view is used to visualize paranasal sinuses :** **AIIMS 1981**
A. AP view B. Towne's view
C. Water's view D. Subment vertical view

56. **The first endoscope was invented by :** **AIIMS 1983**
A. Phillip Bozzini B. Gustav Killian
C. Dulius Bruch D. Warner Forssman

57. **Estimation of fetal maturity by biparietal sonic measurement is accurate within :** **DNB 1984**
A. 3 - 7 days B. 7 - 10 days
C. 10 - 15 days D. 14 - 20 days
E. 3 - 4 weeks

Ans. 36. C 37. C 38. C 39. A 40. D 41. A 42. C 43. C 44. B 45. C
46. C 47. B 48. B 49. C 50. D 51. C 52. A 53. C 54. D 55. C
56. A 57. B

58. **On a mammogram following may be seen except : AIIMS 1983**
A. Calcification is commonly widely distributed in sclerosing adenosis.
B. Fibroadenomas can be seen without radiologically demonstrateable calcification.
C. Fine irregular calcification is seen in intraduct carcinoma.
D. Large, flake-like, irregular calcification is seen in intraduct carcinoma.
E. Eggshell calcification is seen in galactoceles.

59. **Most serious complication of myelogram is : AI 1999**
A. Allergy
B. Transient neurological deficit
C. Headache
D. Arachnoiditis

60. **Most commonly used CT scanners at present are : AMU 1989**
A. First generation B. Second generation
C. Third generation D. Fourth generation

61. **For chromocystoscopy, dye used is : AMC 1984, 89**
A. Sodium iodine B. Lipoidal
C. Indigocarmine D. Conary

62. **Intravenous cholangiogram is not useful if serum bilirubin is above : Delhi 1983, 86; AMC 1984**
A. 1.5 mg % B. 5.3 mg %
C. 10 mg % D. 12.5 mg%

63. **Intravenous pyelography is done with precaution in patients with : Delhi 1985, 86; AMC 1985, 89**
A. Renal calculi B. SLE
C. Multiple myeloma D. Hypertension

64. **Excretory urography should be cautiously performed in case of : AMU 1986**
A. Leukaemia B. Neuroblastoma
C. Bone secondaries D. Multiple myeloma

65. **Oral cholecystography is unlikely to be successful in patients with serum bilirubin above : Delhi 1982, 84; AIIMS 1984**
A. 5 mg% B. 3 mg %
C. 1.5 mg% D. 0.5 mg%

66. **Sonographic appearance of renal transplant rejection is : AIIMS 1982**
A. Increased echogenicity
B. Collection of fluid around kidney
C. Decrease in size of kidney
D. Increased kidney size

67. **Lymphangiography is useful in : AMC 1986**
A. Lymphomas B. Gynaecological
C. Testicular tumours D. All of the above

68. **Contrast material used in the diagnosis of esophageal atresia is : PGI 1987, 88**
A. Barium swallow B. Gastrograffin
C. Conary D. Dianosil

69. **Dye used in IV cholangiography is : PGI 1985, 88**
A. Dianosil B. Conary
C. Biligraffi D. Myodil

70. **Following are seen in mammography except : AP 1995**
A. Translucency
B. Opacity of a cyst
C. Impalpable breast carcinoma in its preclinical stage
D. Demonstrate soft tissue architecture of the breast

71. **Hyperpyrexia in oncology means : PGI 1997**
A. Infection
B. Production of heat within tumour due to radiotherapy
C. ↑ BMR
D. Any of the above

72. **Diagnosis of fetal maturity by ultrasound is best done by : Delhi 1996**
A. Biparietal diameter B. Length of radius
C. Diameter of thorax D. Abdominal girth

73. **MRI is better than CT in all aspects except : Kerala 1996**
A. MRI is more sensitive to pick up smaller lesion.
B. MRI can differentiate between grey & white matter.
C. MRI can pick-up calcified lesions better than CT.
D. MRI can pick-up spinal lesions better.
E. None of the above.

74. **For ascending urethrogram the dye-amount used is ——ml : DNB 1995**
A. 5-10 B. 10-20
C. 20-30 D. 30-40

75. **Father of computerised tomography is : BHU 1996**
A. Sutton B. Hounsfield
C. Curie D. Williams

76. **In a patient with lymphoedema, following may result from lymphangiography with lipoidal except : PGI 1995**
A. Lymphangitis B. Pulm. oedema
C. Cerebral oedema D. - in oedema

77. **The modality that cannot be used in a patient with pacemaker is : Rajasthan 1994**
A. X-ray B. USG
C. CT scan D. NMR

78. **Ultrasonography on umbilical artery signifies : PGI 1997**
A. Heart beat B. Gestational age
C. Foetal weight D. None of the above

Ans.									
58. D	59. D	60. C	61. C	62. B	63. C	64. D	65. A	66. D	67. D
68. D	69. C	70. A	71. B	72. A	73. C	74. D	75. B	76. D	77. D
78. A									

79. USG in ectopic pregnancy is best done : PGI 1997
A. Preabdominal B. Transvaginal
C. Intra-abdominal D. Not useful

80. On USG, in non-immune hydrops foetalis, following are seen except : AIIMS 1997
A. Skin edema B. Large placenta
C. Ascites D. Pericardial effusion

81. Pantomogram is useful in visualization of following except : JIPMER 1998
A. Dental cyst
B. Caries
C. Temporo-mandibular joint
D. Dislocation atlas

82. MRI is contraindicated in patients with : JIPMER 1998
A. Cochlear implants
B. Sensitivity to dye
C. Intracranial haemorrhage
D. Coma

83. All of the following statements about ultrasound are true except : MAHE 1996
A. Medical ultrasound uses the range of 0.1-0.5 MHz.
B. The velocity of sound is greater in bone than that in soft tissue.
C. Ultrasound is generated by the effect of electricity on a ceramic crystal.
D. A sector scanner may involve single or multiple transducers.

84. A crown-rump length of 120 mm corresponds to a gestational age of : MAHE 1996
A. 8 weeks B. 14 weeks
C. 20 weeks D. 26 weeks

85. Which of the following is not a radiological change in mucopolysacharidosis : Delhi 1998
A. J-shaped sella turcica
B. Spatulate ribs
C. Anterior breaking of the vertebra
D. Genu varum

86. 'Wave' or 'Sail' sign is seen in : DNB 1997
A. Craniopharyngioma B. Fourth ventricular cyst
C. Thymic hyperplasia D. Hydatid in lung

87. Radiological investigation to be preferred in a patient with predominantly claSsified intracerebral lesion is: Orissa 1999
A. Digital substraction angiography
B. Magnetic Resonance Imaging
C. Cranial computed tomography
D. Computerised skull X-ray

88. A small contracted and elevated caecum, on barium meal follow through examination is seen most commonly in : Orissa 1999
A. Ulcerative colitiis
B. Crohn's disease
C. Peutz-Jegher's syndrome
D. Chronic ileo-caecal tuberculosis

89. Acute erosive gastritis is best diagnosed by : Orissa 1999
A. Gastric analysis B. Endoscopy
C. Barium meal studies D. Capsule biopsy

90. A given weight of lead is more effective for gamma smelang below 1 M.V. because it has : Orissa 1999
A. Greater strength B. Lesser C1 volume
C. Greater volume D. Higher Atomic number

91. The best X-ray view for the evaluation of a scaphoid fracture is : AI 1988
A. Anteroposterior B. Lateral
C. Oblique D. Axial

92. Trismus in oral cancer patients is severe who was treated with : Karnataka 1999
A. Surgery and radiotherapy
B. Chemotherapy alone
C. Surgery alone
D. Not related to treatment

93. In head and neck cancer patients, good oral hygiene is essential during radiotherapy : Karnataka 1999
A. True
B. Only during chemotherapy
C. Only during surgery
D. Combination treatment with chemotherapy and surgery

94. Slice of tissue using X-rays is : PGI 1999
A. Tomography B. Mammography
C. Contrast studies D. All of the above

95. Which one of the following is not an absolute indication of X-ray of the hip: AIIMS 1999
A. Breech presentation
B. One leg shortened
C. Infantile hip instability
D. Family h/o CDH

96. Radioactivity was discovered by Becqueral in : TN 1999
A. 1796 B. 1896
C. 1901 D. 1946

97. Best investigation for Ileocolic intessusception : TN 1999
A. Barium enema B. Plain X-ray
C. Ultrasound D. CT

98. Occipitomental view of PNS is : Kerala 1999
A. Towne's view B. Water's view
C. Caldwell view D. All of the above

99. I125 is : Kerala 1999
A. Free radicals
B. Low energy photons
C. Low linear transfer radiation
D. High energy photons

Ans.										
	79. A	80. D	81. B	82. A	83. A	84. B	85. D	86. C	87. C	88. D
	89. B	90. D	91. C	92. A	93. D	94. A	95. A	96. B	97. A	98. B
	99. B									

100. The ratio-isotope used for lymph node scanning is : UPSC 2000
A. Technetium 99 B. Iodine 131
C. Phosphorus 32 D. Gallium 67

101. CT Scan is useful in lesions of : Delhi 2000
A. Optic nerve B. V-nerve
C. Trachlear D. Hypoglossal nerve

102. Contrast used in CT is : Delhi 2000
A. Gadolinum B. Technetium
C. Iodine D. Chromium

103. Non-viable part of myocardium are diagnosed by all except : UP 2000
A. Tc99 scintigraphy
B. Thallium scintigraphy
C. Positron emission tomography
D. Standard CT

104. Karnofsky scale is applied in : Kerala 2000
A. Measurement of the size of Tumors.
B. Measurement of the surface area.
C. Evaluation of patients before treatment.
D. Dosage measurement of chemotherapy.
E. Palliative treatment of cancer.

105. All the following are true about iodinated intravascular contrast media except : Kerala 2000
A. They are used in digital subtraction angiography.
B. They are radio opaque.
C. They can cause anaphylactic reactions.
D. They are used in magnetic resonance imaging.
E. They are excreted mainly by the kidneys.

106. Absolute contraindication for IVP is : AI 1992
A. Idiosyncrasy to iodine B. Multiple myeloma
C. Raised blood urea D. All of the above

107. Best imaging modality in patients with breast implants is : Delhi 2001
A. MRI scan B. CT scan
C. Mammography D. Radionuclide scan

108. High resolution CT is the investigation of choice for : Kerala 2001
A. Cystic fibrosis B. Bronchiectasis
C. Pulm. embolism D. T.B.

109. Three dimensional picture of biological molecule is possible by : Rohtak 2001
A. CAT scan B. X-ray crystallography
C. Electron microscope D. NMR imaging

110. USG probe is made-up of : Maharashtra 2000
A. Barium B. Quartz
C. Sodium Iodide D. Diamond

111. MIBG scan is specifically used for diagnosis of : CMC 2001
A. Adrenal tumors B. Pancreatic tumors
C. Parathyroid tumors D. Thyroid tumors
E. Gall bladder tumor

112. Dye for myelography is injected in which space ? Maharashtra 2002
A. Subdural B. Epidural
C. Subarachnoid D. Extradural

113. All electromagnetic waves have same : A.P. 2002
A. Velocity B. Frequency
C. Wavelength D. Velocity & frequency

114. 'Rapid sequence excretory urography' is used in : A.P. 2002
A. Bladder schistosomiasis
B. Urethral calculus
C. Renal transplant rejection
D. Vesicoureteric reflux

115. 'Multiple gated" Radionuclide cardiac scan is used for : A.P. 2002
A. Testing drug toxicity on myocardium
B. Myocardial perfusion assessment
C. Testing verticular function
D. Detecting myocardial aneurysm

116. In a male fetus, ultrasound identification of bilateral hydronephrosis and bladder dilatation is diagnostic of : UPSC 2002
A. Polycystic kidney disease
B. Multicystic dysplastic kidney
C. Uteropelvic junction obstruction
D. Posterior urethral valve syndrome

117. High-resolution CT of the lung is a specialized CT technique for greater detail of lung parenchyma and it utilizes : AIIMS 2002
A. Special lung filters
B. Thick collimation
C. Bone algorithm for image reconstruction
D. Large field of view

118. X-rays are produced when : AIIMS 2002
A. Electron beam strikes the nucleus of the atom.
B. Electron beam strikes the anode.
C. Electron beam reacts with the electromagnetic field.
D. Electron beam strikes the cathode.

119. High resolution computed tomography of the chest is the ideal modality for evaluating : AI 2003
A. Pleural effusion B. Interstitial lung diseasc
C. Lung mass D. Mediastinal adenopathy

120. A 25 years old man presented with fever, cough, expectoration, and breathlessness of 2 months duration. Contrast enhanced computed tomography of chest showed bilateral upper lobe fibrotic lesions and mediastinum has enlarged necrotic nodes with peripheral rim enhancement. Which one of the following is the most probable diagnosis : AI 2003
A. Sarcoidosis B. Tuberculosis
C. Lymphoma D. Silicosis

Ans. 100. D 101. A 102. C 103. D 104. C 105. D 106. D 107. A 108. B 109. B 110. B 111. A 112. C 113. A 114. D 115. A 116. D 117. C 118. B 119. B 120. B

121. Which of the following is the best choice to evaluate radiologically a posterior fossa tumor : AI 2003

A. CT Scan B. MRI
C. Angiography D. Myelography

122. A patient is suspected to have vestibular Schwannoma. The investigation of choice for its diagnosis is: AI 2004

A. Contrast enhanced CT scan
B. Gadolinium enhanced MRI
C. SPECT
D. PET Scan

123. In scurvy all of the following radiological signs are seen except : AI 2004

A. Pelican spur
B. Soap bubble appearance
C. Zone of demarcation near epiphysis
D. Frenkel's line

124. Which of the following is not an indication of RT in Pleomorphic adenoma of parotid : AI 2004

A. Involvement of deep lobe
B. 2nd histologically benign recurrence
C. Microscopically positive margins
D. Malignant transformation

125. Which one of the following radioisotope is not used as permanent implant : AI 2005

A. Iodine - 125 B. Palladium - 103
C. Gold - 198 D. Caesium - 137

126. The four points of probe placement in Focussed Abdominal Sonogram for Trauma (FAST) in blunt thoraco-abdominal trauma are: Karnataka 2004

A Epigastrium, → hypochondrium, (L) Lower chest, hypo-gastrium.
B Epigastrium, → and (L) Hypochondria → Iliac fossa.
C Epigastrium, → and (L) Lumbar regions, hypogastrium.
D Hypogastrium, → and (L) Lumbar regions, → lower chest.

127. Which one of the following conditions is diagnosed by Tc 99 Pertechnetate Scintigraphy : UPSC 2004

A. Pharyngeal diverticulum
B. Duodenal diverticulum
C. Meckel's diverticulum
D. Colonic diverticulum

128. The most sensitive imaging modality for diagnosing ureteric stones in a patients with acute colic is : AI 2005

A. X-ray KUB region
B. Ultrasonogram
C. Non-contrast CT scan of the abdomen
D. Contrast enhanced CT scan of the abdomen

129. There is no radiation in the following investigation : Karnataka 2005

A. CT scan B. Fluoroscopy
C. MRI Scan D. Mammography

130. In Radionuclide imaging the most useful radio pharmaceutical for skeletal imaging is : AI 2005

A. Gallium 67 (67 Ga)
B. Technetium-sulphur-colloid (99mTc-Sc)
C. Technetium-99m (99m(Tc)
D. Technetium-99m linked to Methylene disphosphonate (99m Tc-MDP)

131. In which one of the following conditions the Sialography is contraindicated : AI 2005

A. Ductal calculus
B. Chronic parotitis
C. Acute parotitis
D. Recurrent sialadenitis

132. Radionuclide used in pheochromocytoma is : COMEDK-2005

A. Radioactive Iodine - I131
B. Technetium pertechnicate
C. Radiolabelled Chromium
D. I123 Meta iodate benzyl guanide

133. With reference to mammography, which one of the following statements is correct ? UPSC 2005

A. A baseline study should be done for all women at age 30.
B. It uses less radiation energy than a chest X-ray.
C. It should be part of the regular follow up of a woman following therapy for unilateral breast cancer.
D. It provides an effective substitute for biopsy of suspicious lesions.

134. PACS in medical imaging stands for : AIIMS 2008

A. Planned archieving common system
B. Planned archiving computerized system
C. Picture archiving and communication system
D. Picture archiving or computerized system

135. Most sensitive investigation for DCIS invasive is : AI 2009

A. Mammography B. USG
C. MRI D. PET

136. On USG diffuse thickening of gall bladder with hyperachoic shadow at neck and comet-tailing is seen in : AI 2009

A. Xanthogranulomatous cholecystitis
B. Adenomyomatosis
C. Adenomyomatous polyps
D. Cholesterol crystals

Ans.									
121. B	122. B	123. B	124. A	125. D	126. A	127. C	128. C	129. C	130. D
131. C	132. D	133. C	134. C	135. C	136. B				

137. Reversible ischemia of the heart is detected by : AIIMS 2009

A. Angiography
B. Thallium^{201}-scan
C. MUGA
D. Resting Echocardiography

138. C1 C2 best seen in : AIIMS 2009

A. Lateral view B. Oblique view
C. AP view D. Odontoid view

139. 'Time of flight' technique employed in : Delhi 2009

A. Spiral CT B. M.R. imaging
C. CT. angiography D. Digital radiography

140. Regarding plain X-ray, which of the following is correct : Delhi 2009

A. Should be done in full expiration
B. Should be centered at umbilicus
C. Erect positions is required for suspected perforation
D. Should only be done empty stomach

141. In which of the following form of imaging, Harmonic imaging is related : Delhi 2009

A. Sonography B. Digital radiography
C. MRCP D. Nuclear imaging

142. Functional is analysis is of kidney is best done by : Delhi 2002, 2009

A. Radio nuclide scanning B. IVP
C. Ultrasound D. MRI

143. X-rays are modified : Delhi 2009

A. Protons B. Electrons
C. Neutrons D. Positrons

Ans. 137. B 138. D 139. B 140. C 141. A 142. A 143. B

EXPLANATIONS OF RADIOIMAGING

1. Ans.— B. Cahoon
2. Ans.— B. Ultrasonic flow detector
3. Ans.— D. Rhese
4. Ans.— B. Fracture patella
5. Ans.— C. Anencephaly
6. Ans.— B. Breast
7. Ans.— D. Better visualization of bone and small calcifications.
8. Ans.— C. Viable from non-viable tissue
9. Ans.— D. Cardiac pacemakers
10. Ans.— D. Position Emission Tomography (PET)
11. Ans.— C. MRI
12. Ans.— D. Brain biopsy
13. Ans.— A. Mild mitral stenosis
14. Ans.— B. X-ray lateral view of neck in extension position.
15. Ans.— B. Collecting Tubules
16. Ans.— D. Soft tissue image of neck
17. Ans.— B. Foetal kidney function
18. Ans.— D. Angiography
19. Ans.— C. Spleen
20. Ans.— D. Adamantinoma
21. Ans.— B. Extrinsic bladder compression
22. Ans.— D. Mento vertical
23. Ans.— B. Bone appears gray
24. Ans.— B. Hodgkin's disease
25. Ans.— A. Renal tumours

    Micturating cystourethrogram is done to demonstrate urethra and bladder neck (in males) and to demonstrate bladder mechanisms, in particular stress incontinence and in children, posterior urethral valves.
26. Ans.— E. Dianosil
27. Ans.— D. Vertebral column
28. Ans.— D. Base of skull view
29. Ans.— B. Mastoid air cells
30. Ans.— B. Recurrent subluxation
31. Ans.— B. CT scan
32. Ans.— D. Full bladder
33. Ans.— C. Cardiovascular malformation

    It is particularly useful in assessment of valvular lesions.
34. Ans.— D. Myodil
35. Ans.— C. 2 int. carotids + 1 vertebral
36. Ans.— C. Dorsal metatarsal vein
37. Ans.— C. Micturating cystogram

    Radioisotop scan using Tc-99 DTPA can also be used.
38. Ans.— C. Electromusical Instruments, England

    It was invented by Geoffery Hounsfield.
39. Ans.— A. Iapanoic acid
40. Ans.— D. Retroperitoneal liposarcoma
41. Ans.— A. Sinuses
42. Ans.— C. Methyglucamine iodipamide
43. Ans.— C. Conary 480
44. Ans.— B. 30 %
45. Ans.— C. Japan
46. Ans.— C. Small bowel enema
47. Ans.— B. Barium sulphate
48. Ans.— B. Bronchiectasis
49. Ans.— C. Post. Ethmoidal
50. Ans.— D. Grey and a white matter differentiation
51. Ans.— C. Salivary glands

    Sialography is performed by injecting either the parotid or submaxillary duct, 1-2 ml of viscous or water soluble contrast medium.
52. Ans.— A. Selective arteriograph
53. Ans.— C. Orbital echography
54. Ans.— D. +20 to +45
55. Ans.— C. Water's view
56. Ans.— A. Phillip Bozzini
57. Ans.— B. 7 - 10 days

58. Ans.— D. Large, flake-like, irregular calcification is seen in intraduct carcinoma.

59. Ans.— D. Arachnoiditis

It is now performed with water soluble low osmolar contrast medium to demonstrate intra or extra medullary tumors, cauda equina, disc prolapse.

60. Ans.— C. Third generation

61. Ans.— C. Indigocarmine

62. Ans.— B. 5.3 mg %

63. Ans.— C. Multiple myeloma

64. Ans.— D. Multiple myeloma

Contraindications also includes proteinuria and diabetics with creatinine more than 2 mg%.

65. Ans.— A. 5 mg%

Dose used is 6 Tablets of 0.5 g 2 hours after evening meals. Bilirubin should be below 5 mg%. Absolutely contraindicated in serious liver disease and relatively contraindicated in peritonitis, post-operative ileus and acute pancreatitis.

66. Ans.— D. Increased kidney size

Tc-99 DTPA is used.

67. Ans.— D. All of the above

68. Ans.— D. Dianosil

69. Ans.— C. Biligraffi

70. Ans.— A. Translucency

71. Ans.— B. Production of heat within tumour due to radiotherapy.

72. Ans.— A. Biparietal diameter

73. Ans.— C. MRI can pick-up calcified lesions better than CT.

74. Ans.— D. 30-40

75. Ans.— B. Hounsfield

76. Ans.— D. - in oedema

77. Ans.— D. NMR

78. Ans.— A. Heart beat

79. Ans.— A. Preabdominal

80. Ans.— D. Pericardial effusion

81. Ans.— B. Caries

82. Ans.— A. Cochlear implants

83. Ans.— A. Medical ultrasound uses the range of 0.1-0.5 MHz.

84. Ans.— B. 14 weeks

85. Ans.— D. Genu varum

86. Ans.— C. Thymic hyperplasia

87. Ans.— C. Cranial computed tomography

88. Ans.— D. Chronic ileo-caecal tuberculosis

89. Ans.— B. Endoscopy

Endoscopy can visualize the changes.

90. Ans.— D. Higher Atomic number

91. Ans.— C. Oblique

PA and oblique views should be taken with ulnar deviation of the hand, together with a lateral.

92. Ans.— A. Surgery and radiotherapy

93. Ans.— D. Combination treatment with chemotherapy and surgery.

94. Ans.— A. Tomography

95. Ans.— A. Breech presentation

96. Ans.— B. 1896

97. Ans.— A. Barium enema

98. Ans.— B. Water's view

99. Ans.— B. Low energy photons

100. Ans.— D. Gallium 67

101. Ans.— A. Optic nerve

102. Ans.— C. Iodine

103. Ans.— D. Standard CT

104. Ans.— C. Evaluation of patients before treatment.

105. Ans.— D. They are used in magnetic resonance imaging.

106. Ans.— D. All of the above

Contraindications also includes proteinuria and diabetics with creatinine more than 2 mg%.

107. Ans.— A. MRI scan

108. Ans.— B. Bronchiectasis

109. Ans.— B. X-ray crystallography

110. Ans.— B. Quartz

111. Ans.— A. Adrenal tumors

112. Ans.— C. Subarachnoid

113. Ans.— A. Velocity

114. Ans.— D. Vesicoureteric reflux

115. Ans.— A. Testing drug toxicity on myocardium

116. Ans.— D. Posterior urethral valve syndrome

117. Ans.— C. Bone algorithm for image reconstruction

118. Ans.— B. Electron beam strikes the anode

119. Ans.— B. Interstitial lung disease

120. Ans.— B. Tuberculosis

121. Ans.— B. MRI

* "PET & MRI are used in surgical on radiosurgical planning to define anatomic relationship of Tumor to critical Brain regions".
* Ghai says "CT evaluates anatomy of supratentorial brain structures reasonably well. Posterior fossa and brain stem structure are not well visualized.

122. Ans.— B. Gadolinium enhanced MRI

Vestibular schwannomas characteristically present as progressive unilateral hearing loss rather than with dizziness or other vestibular symptoms.

- MRI with gadolinium contrast is superior to CT scan.

123. Ans.— B. Soap bubble appearance

Scurvy

- Earliest signs are seen at the knees.
- Osteoporosis (usually the only sign seen in adults) Loss of epiphyseal density with a pencil-thin cortex (Wimberger's sign).
- Metaphyseal lucency (Trummerfeld zone)
- Metaphyseal corner fractures through the weekened lucent of the metaphysis (Pelkan spurs) resulting in cupping of the metaphysis.
- Periosteal reaction due to subperiosteal haematoma.

124. Ans.— A. Involvement of deep lobe

125. Ans.— D. Caesium - 137

* Image-Guided Brachytherapy
  - CT Guided 198 A4 (Gold) implants for the treatment of rectal carcinoma.
  - Sonographically guided 125I and 103 Pd implant for the treatment of Prostate Cancer.
  - Real time treatment planning in the procedure room using a laptop-based treatment planning computer.
  - This procedure allows radiation oncologist to view the dose as the 103 Pd, 125I or 198 A4 seeds are implanted and to adjust the planned location of each seed in light of this information.

Future plans are to combien real time treatment planning dosimetry with CT-guided and fluoroscopic verification of seed placement for permanent prostate implants

126. Ans.— A. Epigastrium →hypochondrium, (L) Lower chest, hypogastrium

127. Ans.— C. Meckel's diverticulum

128. Ans.— C. Non-contrast CT scan of the abdomen

* The test of choice at most centers for diagnosing an acute stone is a non-contrast, helical CT scan.
* All stones, regardless of composition, are visualised on CT scan with the exception of a small percentage of indinavir stones. Indinavir stones form in HIV-positive patients treated with the protease inhibitor indinavir sulphate.
* Though plain X-ray abdomen and pelvis is the simplest way to obtain, radiolucent stones such as uric acid stones and cystine stones may not be visualised.

129. Ans.— C. MRI Scan

130. Ans.— D. Technetium-99m linked to Methylene disphosphonate (99m Tc-MDP)

"Technetium-99m methylene diphosphonate (99mTc-MDP) is the agent of choice, since it renders a low radiation dose, a convenient half life for clinical use, and monoenergetic 140-KeV photon ideal for current imaging devices."

131. Ans.— C. Acute parotitis

"Dialography is contraindicated for clinically active infection, as it will often spread the infection retrograde into the gland. Additionally, as acute sialoadenitis is already painful, the patient will not tolerate the additional discomfort of the retrograde pressure injection required for an adequate sialogram."

Indications for Sialography :

1. Detection or confirmation of small parotid or submandibular gland sialolith or foreign bodies (calcified/non-calcified)
2. Evaluation of the extent of irreversible ductal damage present as a result of infection

3. Differentiation of disease such as chronic sialoadenitis/parotitis.
4. Evaluation of fistular, stricture, diverticular, communicating cysts, ductal trauma.
5. Dilating procedure for mild ductal stenosis.

132. Ans.— D. I123 Meta iodate benzyl guanide.

Patients with metallic Gazettes (Pacemakers, valves, stents, cochlear implants etc.) are not taken up for MRI.

133. Ans.— C. It should be part of the regular follow up of a woman following therapy for unilateral breast cancer.

134. Ans.— C Picture archiving and communication system

* PACS or picture archiving and communication system are computerized network dedicated to the image acquisition, storage, transportation and display.

135. Ans.— C. MRI

* While MRI has demonstrated variable specificity, the reported sensitivities of this technique for the visualization of invasive breast cancer in the diagnostic setting has approached 100% in several studies.

136. Ans.— B. Adenomyomatosis

The hyperplastic cholecystoses :

Hyperplastic cholecystoses is a group of disorders of the gall bladder characterized by excessive proliferation of normal tissue components. It includes cholecystitis glandularis proliferans.

137. Ans.— B. Thallium^{201} scan

When the resting ECG is abnormal (e.g., pre-excitation syndrome >1 mm of resting ST-segment depression, left bundle branch block, paced ventricular rhythm), information gained from an exercise test can be enhanced by stress myocardial radionuclide perfusion imaging after the intravenous administration of thallium 201 or technetium 99m (^{99m}Tc) seastamibi during exercise (or a pharmacologic) stress.

Thallium Scan :

* ^{201}Tl (thallium) was the first isotope used for this purpose.
* It has been largely replaced by 99mTc, which has a higher photon energy and shorter half-life, permitting the injection of larger doses resulting in scans of higher quality.
* To technetium-labelled myocardium perfusion agents are in common use- tetrofosmin and sestamibi.
* Like thallium, both tetrofosmin and sestamibi distribute to the myocardium in relation to blood flow, and their uptake requires an intact cell membrane are bond within the cell in a nearly irreversible fashion. As a result, these agents must generally be injected twice— once at rest and once during stress.

138. Ans.— D. Odontoid view

Fractures of the odontoid Process or Dens

* Fractures of the odontoid process are usually transversely oriented and situated at the base of the odontoid. There may be anterior or posterior displacement, depending upon the nature of the injuring force.

139. Ans.— B. M.R. imaging

140. Ans.— C. Erect positions is required for suspected perforation

141. Ans.— A. Sonography

142. Ans.— A. Radio nuclide scanning

143. Ans.— B. Electrons

9

MCQ's OF MISCELLANEOUS

What is important in Miscellaneous

Named Signs, Diagnostic features of important common diseases, Recent advances

1. **Causes of nasal bone erosion include all except : AMU 1983**
A. Sarcoidosis B. Wegener's granuloma
C. Bismuth poisoning D. Cocaine addiction
2. **The useful diagnostic aid in trophoblastic tumour is : AMU 1985**
A. Ultrasonography B. HCG titre estimation
C. Clinical examination D. Amniography
3. **The treatment of choice in nasopharyngeal fibroma is : Delhi 1989, 92; AI 1989**
A. Radiotherapy
B. Hormone therapy
C. Surgical removal
D. Surgical removal followed by radiotherapy
4. **Patient with Cushing's disease may show in chest : DNB 1991**
A. Pleural fluid
B. Hilar adenopathy
C. Small heart
D. Widening of mediastinum
5. **Which is not demonstrtable in Cushing's syndrome : AIIMS 1985**
A. Osteosclerosis
B. Abnormal callus formation
C. Osteoporosis
D. Pathological fractures
6. **The osseous manifestation of acute leukaemia is/are : PGI 1985**
A. Periosteal reaction
B. Osteolytic lesions
C. Diffuse demineralisation
D. Osteosclerotic reaction
E. All are true
7. **The following are not manifestations of neurofibromatosis : PGI 1985**
A. Sclerosis of the orbital walls
B. Osteomalacia
C. Hypertrophy of a limb
D. Renal artery aneurysms
E. Optic nerve glioma
8. **On a lateral cervical radiograph widening of prevertebral soft tissues can occur in all except : AIIMS 1981**
A. Haemophilia B. Trauma
C. Laryngomalacia D. Tuberculosis
E. Sickle cell disease
9. **Thesaurosis is a disease said by some to be related to : AIIMS 1985**
A. Molding of copper tube
B. Resins in hair spray
C. Inhalation of barium dust
D. Inoenophiles
E. Male singers
10. **'Sausage digit' is typically seen in : DNB 1996**
A. Rheumatoid arthritis B. Leprosy
C. Psoriasis D. Osteoarthritis
11. **Hilar and mediastinal node enlargement in Hodgkin's disease is most often : Delhi 1981**
A. Unilateral
B. Primarily hilar
C. Bilateral and symmetrical
D. Bilateral and asymmetrical
12. **A child showing failure to grow, anaemia, and wooly moutheaten appearance of the long bone metaphysis and skull with widened epiphyseal lines probably suffers from : PGI 1983**
A. Syphilis B. Renal rickets
C. Rickets D. Scurvy
13. **Aniline dyes are commonly the etiological agents for carcinoma of : AMU 1986; AI 1990**
A. Thyroid B. Kidney
C. Prostate D. Urinary bladder
14. **Primary anomaly in Klippel-Feil syndrome is : AMU 1986**
A. Torticolits B. Fusion
C. Absence D. Segmentation

Ans.	1. C	2. A	3. C	4. D	5. A	6 E	7. A	8. E	9. B	10. C
	11. D	12. B	13. D	14. B						

15. **'Honey Comb' appearance on X-ray may be seen in the following except : Bihar 1989**
A. Osteoclastoma B. Paget's disease
C. Fibrous dysplasia D. Adamantinoma

16. **Hamman-Rich syndrome is : AIIMS 1986**
A. Fibrosing alveolitis
B. Rapidly progressive interstitial pulmonary fibrosis
C. Recurrent spontaneous pneumothoraxes
D. Central mediastinal adenopathy

17. **Lymphangiomyomatosis in characterized by all of the following except : AIIMS 1985**
A. Postmenopausal women
B. Recurrent chylous pleural effusions
C. Ascites
D. Recurrent spontaneous pneumothoraxes

18. **Weightlessness in space travel causes : AIIMS 1989**
A. Difficulty in deglutition
B. Decreased motility of colon
C. Arterial hypotension
D. Demineralisation of bone

19. **Wegner granulomatosis is a triad of the diseases of following except : PGI 1989**
A. Lung B. Renal
C. Liver D. Sinus

20. **Egg shell calcification in hilar nodes may be seen in : AIIMS 1986**
A. Silicosis B. Sarcoidosis
C. Treated lymphoma D. All of the above

21. **'Chevron sign' is seen in : DNB 1998**
A. Fluorosis B. Achondroplasia
C. Perthes disease D. Paget's disease

22. **'Gloved-tree appearance in chest X-ray is seen in : DNB 1998**
A. Pneumoconiosis B. Histoplasmosis
C. Bronchiectasis D. Interstitial lung disease

23. **'Hampton's line' is seen in : AIIMS 1997**
A. Scurvy
B. Hypoparathyroidism
C. Gastric ulcer
D. Patent vitellointestinal duct

24. **Schistosomal infection produces all except : AMU 1988**
A. Polypoidal lesion in the distal colon
B. Paraplegia
C. Pulmonary arterial hypertension
D. Oesophageal varices
E. Hilar-lymphadenopathy

25. **On erect chest X-ray, or left decubitus abdominal films, it is possible to demonstrate as little as ----- ml gas in abdomen. AIIMS 1997**
A. 1 B. 5
C. 10 D. 50

26. **In congenital syphilis, Saber tibia results due to : DNB 1997**
A. Periostitis B. Diaphysitis
C. Metaphysitis D. Osteomyelitis

27. **Following are radiological features of scurvy except : AIIMS 1997**
A. Cupping of metaphysis
B. Metaphyseal lucency
C. Hyperparathyroidism
D. Osteoporosis

28. **True about Syringomyelia is following except : AIIMS 1982**
A. Produces neurological signs in upper and lower limbs.
B. Commonly involves the dorsal columns.
C. Is associated with a scoliosis.
D. Is commonly associated with Arnold Chiari malformation.

29. **'Pencil tip' deformity is seen in : PGI 1994**
A. Carcinoma pharynx B. Achalasia Cardia
C. Barrett's oesophagus D. None of the above

30. **Leather bottle appearance on chest X-ray is seen in : AMU 1986**
A. Pericardial effusion
B. Pulmonary oedema
C. Constrictive pericarditis
D. Pulm. artery hypertension

31. **Radio-immunoassay of CEA in blood is found to be positive in following except : DNB 1992**
A. Diabetes mellitus
B. Emphysema
C. Alcoholic cirrhosis
D. Colorectal carcinoma
E. None of the above

32. **Term 'vanishing tumor' is used for : AIIMS 1981**
A. Organized emphysema
B. Loculated pleural effusion
C. Neurofibromatosis
D. Hydatid cyst

33. **To distinguish AVM (arterio-venous malformation) from neoplasm, the best is : AMU 1991**
A. Fundus
B. EEG
C. Cerebral angiography
D. CT scanning

34. **Which of the following ultrasound marker is associated with greatest increased risk for Trisomy 21 in fetus : AI 2005**
A. Echogenic foci in heart
B. Hyperechogenic bowel
C. Choroid plexus cysts
D. Nuchal edema

Ans.										
	15. C	16. B	17. A	18. D	19. C	20. D	21. B	22. C	23. C	24. E
	25. A	26. A	27. A	28. C	29. D	30. A	31. E	32. B	33. C	34. D

35. Ca breast is not discovered in mammography in young woman due to : AI 2009

A. Dense glandular tissue
B. Fat replaces glandular tissue
C. Loose tissue
D. Thick overlying skin in young

36. Which of the following contain Fat on mammography: AI 2009

A. Traumatic cyst
B. Fibroadenoma
C. Keratosis
*D. Galactocele

37. Prunning of vessels is seen in : AI 2009

A. Lung tumor
B. Primary Pulmonary hypertension
C. Chronic Bronchitis
D. Pulmonary infections

Ans. **35. A** **36. A** **37. B**

EXPLANATIONS OF MISCELLANEOUS

1. Ans.— C. Bismuth poisoning
2. Ans.— A. Ultrasonography
3. Ans.— C. Surgical removal

   Radiotherapy may help in decreasing vascularity before surgery. Transpalatal approach of Wilson is usually used.
4. Ans.— D. Widening of mediastinum
5. Ans.— A. Osteosclerosis
6. Ans.— E. All are true
7. Ans.— A. Sclerosis of the orbital walls
8. Ans.— E. Sickle cell disease
9. Ans.— B. Resins in hair spray
10. Ans.— C. Psoriasis
11. Ans.— D. Bilateral and asymmetrical
12. Ans.— B. Renal rickets
13. Ans.— D. Urinary bladder

    Benzidine is most often implicated. Other carcinogens include arsenic (lung, skin, liver), asbestos (mesothelium, lung), Benzene (leukemia), Chromium compounds (lung), Radiation (mining, dial painting cause cancers at numerous locations), mustard gas (lung) polycyclic hydrocarbons (lung, skin), vinyl chloride (angiosarcoma of liver).
14. Ans.— B. Fusion
15. Ans.— C. Fibrous dysplasia
16. Ans.— B. Rapidly progressive interstitial pulmonary fibrosis.
17. Ans.— A. Postmenopausal women
18. Ans.— D. Demineralisation of bone

    It is a cause of osteoporosis.
19. Ans.— C. Liver
20. Ans.— D. All of the above

    It is most commonly seen in silicosis.
21. Ans.— B. Achondroplasia

    There may also be trident hand, ball in socket epiphysis, champagne glass pelvis and gibbus.
22. Ans.— C. Bronchiectasis
23. Ans.— C. Gastric ulcer

    Hampton's line is 1 mm thin straight lucent line traversing the orifice of ulcer niche (seen in profile view with little gastric distension). There may also be Haudek niche in benign gastric ulcer. In malignant gastric ulcer, Carman meniscus sign and Kirkilin meniscus complex are seen.
24. Ans.— E. Hilar-lymphadenopathy
25. Ans.— A. 1
26. Ans.— A. Periostitis
27. Ans.— A. Cupping of metaphysis
28. Ans.— C. Is associated with a scoliosis
29. Ans.— D. None of the above
30. Ans.— A. Pericardial effusion
31. Ans.— E. None of the above
32. Ans.— B. Loculated pleural effusion
33. Ans.— C. Cerebral angiography
34. Ans.— D. Nuchal edema

    Likelihood ratios for isolated soft marker for Down's syndrome.

Sonographic Findings	*Likelihood Ratio*
1. Nuchal fold 6 mm or more	19
2. Echogenic bowel	5.5
3. Short Femur	2.3
4. Mild renal pelvic dilatation	1.5

* Sonographic scoring system for the detection of trisomy 21.

Sonographic Findings	Score
1. Major defect	2
2. Nuchal fold 6 mm or more	2
3. Short Femur	1
4. Short Humerus	1
5. Mild renal pelvic dilatation	1
6. Echogenic bowel	1

Features with a score of 2 or more are considered at high risk for Down's syndrome.

* **Thickening of the soft tissues at the back of the neck is a useful ultrasound sign in Down Syndrome (approx 16% of Fetuses with Down's syndrome).**
* **A thickness of 6 mm or more is considered abnormal at 16-20 weeks gestation 2nd trisomy 21 is present in 20-40% of fetuses.**
* **Soft markers for Down's syndrome (Minor Findings).**
  1. **Short Femur or Humerus**
  2. **Echogenic bowel**
  3. **Mild renal pelvic dilatation**
  4. **Echogenic foci in Heart**
  5. **Clinodactyly of Fifth Finger and Sandal gap.**
  - **Each marker is present in 1-5% of all pregnancies.**
  * **Now the answer is obvious from the above facts (i.e. choice '4').**

35. Ans.— A. Dense glandular tissue

* **The young woman's breast contains a large proportion of glandular tissue which appears as soft-tissue density on the mammogram in older woman. When involution of the glandular tissue has occurred, most of the breast tissue appears of fatty density.**

36. Ans.— A. Traumatic cyst and Galactocele

and D. Differential diagnosis of fat containing Breast lesions :

* **Lipoma**
* **Oil cyst**
* **Galactocele**
* **Hamartoma**
* **Traumatic cyst**

37. Ans.— B. Primary Pulmonary hypertension

Pulmonary arterial hypertension is recognized by enlargement of the main pulmonary artery and central pulmonary vessels with peripheral vessel pruning.

REVIEW PAPER-I

(Based on Difficult & Important MCQ's)

1. Persistence of canal of Kovalevski can lead to :
A. Sacrococygeal teratoma
B. Neurenteric cyst
C. Sacral agenesis
D. Sacral cyst

2. Candy cane appearance of small GI obstruction is best seen in ——— position.
A. Erect B. Supine
C. Prone D. Lateral

3. Candle drippings in brain are seen in :
A. Toxoplasmosis B. TBM
C. Tuberous sclerosis D. Neurocysticercosis

4. Tear drop fracture is seen in —— vertebra :
A. C1 B. C2
C. C4 D. C7

5. Rolando fracture is seen in :
A. Calcaneum B. Talus
C. Thumb D. Little finger

6. Caroli disease is characterized by following features except :
A. Portal hypertension
B. Associated medullary sponge kidney
C. Recurrent abdominal pain
D. Calculi in dilated ductus

7. Aortic dissection involving ascending aorta only is —— type.
A. De Bakey-I B. De Bakey-II
C. De Bakey-III D. Standard type-B

8. Absence of pars membrancea in trachea leads to —— shape.
A. Inverted-T B. Napkin ring
C. Carrot D. Any of the above

9. Urinoma is a :
A. Tumor B. Stone
C. True cyst D. Pseudocyst

10. 'Celery-stalk sign is seen in :
A. Diphtheria B. Rubella
C. Sarcoidosis D. Scheuermann disease

11. 'Cervix sign' is seen in :
A. Carcinoma uterus
B. Duodenal atresia
C. Hypertrophic Pyloric stenosis
D. Hirschsprung disease

12. Chamberlain line is a line between roof of palate to posterior part of :
A. Foramen magnum B. Axis vertebra
C. C3 vertebra D. C7 vertebra

13. Coke bottle sign is seen in :
A. Haemangioma of orbit
B. Norrie disease
C. Grave's disease
D. Toxocara Endophthalmitis

14. Cobblestone appearance of bile ducts is seen in :
A. Cholesterosis B. Sclerositing cholangitis
C. Pyogenic cholangitis D. Bile duct diverticulum

15. Cobblestoning may be seen in :
A. Candidiasis of esophagus
B. Brunner gland hyperplasia
C. Burkitt lymphoma
D. Ca oesophagus

16. Fleischner lines are commonly associated with :
A. Bronchiectasis B. Bronchial adenoma
C. Pleural effusion D. Ca lung

17. Henry K. Pancoast (who described pancoast tumor) was a :
A. Surgeon B. Anaesthesist
C. Physician D. Radiologist

18. Shaver's disease is a form of :
A. Berryliosis B. Silicosis
C. Aspergillosis D. Pulmonary eosinophilia

19. Convolutional markings in the newborn represent :
A. Rickets B. Cretinism
C. Craniolacunia D. Craniosynostosis

20. Metastatic tumors which may present as subarachnoid haemorrhage are following except :
A. Malignant melanoma B. Choriocarcinoma
C. Ca breast D. Hypernephroma

Ans.										
	1. B	2. A	3. C	4. B	5. C	6. A	7. B	8. B	9. D	10. B
	11. C	12. A	13. C	14. B	15. B	16. D	17. D	18. B	19. C	20. C

21. Collar button ulcers in colon are seen in :
A. Typhoid B. Diverticulitis
C. Amoebiasis D. Ulcerative colitis

22. Double line sign is seen in :
A. Perthes disease B. Fluorosis
C. Osteomalacia D. Osteoclastoma

23. In asomia there is agenesis of vertebral :
A. Body B. Pedicle
C. Arch D. None of the above

24. Myxoglobulosis is a variant of :
A. Meconium ileus B. Mesenteric ischemia
C. Megacolon D. Mucocele appendix

25. "Garland" blush on MRI/CECT is typically seen in :
A. Aging hematoma B. Glioblastoma
C. Meningioma D. Craniopharyngioma

26. Comet tail lung lesion is seen in :
A. Sarcoidosis B. Asbestosis
C. Aspergillosis D. Histoplasmosis

27. Pseudokidney sign on ultrasound is seen in :
A. Duodenum diverticulum
B. Intussusception
C. Ischaemic colitis
D. Ladd bands

28. Heerfordt syndrome is characterized by all except :
A. Chronic sinusitis B. Uveitis
C. Facial nerve paralysis D. Parotid enlargement

29. In renal tuberculosis following findings are true except :
A. Beaded ureter B. Corkscrew ureter
C. Pipestem ureter D. Dropping lily ureter

30. Grow foot sign may be seen in :
A. Acute pancreatitis B. Pseudocyst Pancreas
C. Cholelithiasis D. Sclerosing cholangitis

31. Colon cut off sign is seen in the following except :
A. Ischaemic colitis B. Colonic obstruction
C. Acute Pancreatitis D. Diverticulosis

32. Delta sign or empty triangle sign in brain is seen in :
A. Venous angioma
B. Vein of Galen aneurysm
C. Venous sinus thrombosis
D. Ventriculitis

33. Kommerell diverticulum is seen in :
A. Aorta B. Oesophagus
C. Duodenum D. Bile duct

34. Hutch diverticulum is seen in :
A. Gall bladder B. Stomach
C. Urinary bladder D. Ileum

35. Triple track sign is seen in :
A. Peutz Jegher syndrome
B. Hypertrophic pyloric stenosis
C. Jejunal atresia
D. Ileocaecal TB

36. Kirklen or mushroom sign is seen in :
A. Achalasia cardia
B. Ca oesophagus
C. Ca stomach
D. Hypertrophic pyloric stenosis

37. Coil-spring appearance of gastric filling defect is seen in :
A. Lymphoma in stomach
B. Acid peptic disease
C. Trichobezoar
D. Jejunogastric intussusception

38. Diamond sign is seen in :
A. Ca oesophagus B. IHPS
C. Bile duct stone D. Renal cell carcinoma

39. Double Halo configuration sign is seen in :
A. Ulcerative colitis B. Ischaemic colitis
C. Crohn's disease D. Cystic fibrosis

40. In Ankylosing spondylitis, pulmonary area most often affected is :
A. Apex B. Middle portion
C. Base D. Hilum

41. Goblet sign or Bergman sign is seen in :
A. Meckle's diverticulitis
B. Renal papillary mucosal mass
C. Idiopathic steatorrhoea
D. TB Mesenteritis

42. Colonic thumb printing may be seen in the following except :
A. Ulcerative colitis
B. Crohn's colitis
C. Localized primary lymphoma
D. None of the above

43. "Apical cup sign" is seen in :
A. Mesothelioma
B. Extrapleural haematoma
C. PDA
D. Supravalvular AS

44. Apple core lesion is seen in —— carcinoma colon.
A. Fungating polypoid B. Annular ulcerating
C. Scirrhous D. Curvilnear

45. 'Whirl sign' on CT scan is seen in :
A. Colonic carcinoma
B. Colonic diverticulosis
C. Colonic volvulus
D. Colitis cystica profunda

46. "Apple peel appearance" on Ba studies is seen in :
A. Mucocele of appendix
B. Midgut Volvulus
C. Muconium peritonitis
D. Mesenteric ischaemia

Ans.										
	21. D	22. A	23. A	24. D	25. B	26. B	27. B	28. A	29. D	30. C
	31. D	32. C	33. A	34. C	35. B	36. D	37. D	38. B	39. C	40. A
	41. B	42. D	43. B	44. B	45. B	46. B				

47. Apple sauce appearance is seen in :
A. Meckel diverticulum B. Meconium ileus
C. TB mesenteritis D. Omental cyst

48. 'B' ring of oesophagus is ——— shaped :
A. W B. U
C. M D. L

49. 'A' ring of oesophagus is located at ——— aspect.
A. Superior B. Middle
C. Inferior D. Any of the above

50. Normal number of folds of jejunum per inch is :
A. 2-4 B. 4-6
C. 6-8 D. 8-10

51. Boxer's fracture is common in —— metacarpal :
A. 1 B. 2
C. 3 D. 5

52. In Gamekeeper thumb or skier's thumb, there is :
A. Fracture B. Tendon injury
C. Ligament injury D. All of the above

53. Breslow's staging is for :
A. Neuroblastoma
B. Ca Gall bladder
C. Malignant melanoma
D. Non-Hodgkin's lymphoma

54. Breus mole is :
A. H. mole
B. Choriocarcinoma
C. Subchorial haemorrhage
D. Submucous fibroid

55. Bubbly bone lesion is seen in the following except :
A. Osteoblastoma B. Aneurysmal bone cyst
C. Fibrous dysplasia D. Rickets

56. Eosinophilic granuloma of GIT is most often seen in :
A. Oesophagus B. Stomach
C. Colon D. None of the above

57. Bullet shaped vertebrae may be seen in :
A. Paget's disease B. Multiple myeloma
C. Achondroplasia D. Osteomalacia

58. Jefferson fracture is seen in ——— vertebra.
A. C1 B. C2
C. C7 D. T4

59. 'Buruli ulcer' is caused by :
A. Trypanosoma B. Schistosomiasis
C. Guinea worm D. Atypical mycobacteria

60. Button sequestrum may be seen in all except :
A. TB
B. Eosinophilic granuloma
C. Radiation
D. None of the above

61. 'Bell and Clapper' deformity is seen in :
A. Gall bladder B. Kidney
C. Testiles D. Ureter

62. 'Spring onion' appearance of distal ureter is seen in :
A. Bladder tumor B. Ureteric calculus
C. Ureterocele D. Pseudoureterocele

63. 'Bird beak deformity' is seen in :
A. Congenital megacolon
B. Hypertrophic pyloric stenosis
C. Achalasia cardia
D. Jejunal atresia

64. "Bird wing or Seal gull" joint configuration is seen in :
A. Rheumatoid arthritis B. Osteoarthritis
C. Paget's disease D. Ochronosis

65. Osteoblastoma of spine is most common in —— spine.
A. Cervical B. Dorsal
C. Lumbar D. Sacral

66. Blueberry Muffin syndrome is seen in :
A. Adenocarcinoma B. Neuroblastoma
C. Osteoblastoma D. Phaeochromocytoma

67. Characteristic symptom of 'Page Kidney' is :
A. Haematuria B. Anuria
C. Hypertension D. Nephrocalcinosis

68. Most common cause of 'Page kidney' is :
A. Blunt trauma
B. Spontaneous haematoma
C. Renal cyst
D. Tumor

69. Weigert Meyer rule is seen in insertion of :
A. Latissimus dorsi B. Spermatic cord
C. Vagus nerve D. Ureter

70. 'Penicilling' or 'autoamputation' of terminal tufts is seen in :
A. SLE B. Scleroderma
C. Diabetes mellitus D. Rheumatoid arthritis

71. Azzopardi tumor is seen in :
A. Pancreas B. Kidney
C. Pineal gland D. Testis

72. Backwash ileitis is seen in :
A. Acute ulcerative colitis
B. Chronic ulcerative colitis
C. Muconium ileus
D. Diverticulosis

73. Multiple 'vacuum' phenomenon is seen in :
A. Osgood Schlatter disease
B. Ochronosis
C. Jaffe-Campanacci syndrome
D. Noonan syndrome

Ans.									
47. B	48. B	49. A	50. B	51. D	52. C	53. C	54. C	55. D	56. B
57. C	58. A	59. D	60. D	61. C	62. D	63. C	64. B	65. B	66. B
67. C	68. B	69. D	70. B	71. D	72. B	73. B			

74. **Cotton wool appearance in Paget's disease is seen in :**
A. Pelvis B. Femur
C. Manubrium D. Skull

75. **"Banana fracture" in Paget's disease is seen on :**
A. Humerus B. Femur
C. Vertebra D. Calcaneum

76. **Luxatio erecta is —— dislocation of shoulder :**
A. Anterior B. Posterior
C. Inferior D. None of the above

77. **Trough sign is seen in ——— dislocation of shoulder.**
A. Anterior B. Posterior
C. Superior D. Inferior

78. **Bankart lesion is fracture of :**
A. Superior glenoid rim B. Inferior glenoid rim
C. Greater tuberosity D. Lesser tuberosity

79. **Barber pole sign seen in midgut volvulus is due to spiraling of :**
A. Sup. mesenteric artery B. Inf. mesenteric artery
C. Sup. mesenteric vein D. Inf. mesenteric vein

80. **Candle flame or Blade of grass lysis" in long bones is seen in :**
A. Perthes disease B. Fluorosis
C. Paget's disease D. Rickets

81. **Craniolacunia regresses after :**
A. 1 month B. 3 months
C. 12 months D. 5 years

82. **Choroid plexus papilloma are most common in :**
A. Third ventricle B. Lateral ventricle
C. IV ventricle D. Cerebropontine angle

83. **Local tracheal displacement in the neck is due most commonly to which of the following:**
A. Enlarged thyroid gland
B. Pulmonary atelectasis
C. Cyst
D. Marked pleural effusion

84. **Which of the following is not applicable in regard to rupture of a main-stem bronchus:**
A. Rupture rarely involves a bronchus distal to the main bronchus.
B. The most common cause is blunt trauma to the anterior chest.
C. Bronchial rupture is more common on the left due to the greater length of the left compared to the right.
D. In view of the frequency of bilateral involvement it is important to evaluate both main-stem bronchi if one is found severed/ruptured.

85. **In the case of blunt trauma to the chest without penetrating injury, which of the following is correct:**
A. Traumatic pneumatoceles require 5-7 days to develop.
B. Cavitating pulmonary hematomas develop rapidly, often within 3 days following injury.
C. Fractured first and second ribs are commonly associated with a ruptured bronchus on the same side.
D. Traumatic pneumatoceles are more common in older patients than younger ones.

86. **Tracheal narrowing as seen by roentgenogram may be due to all of the following except :**
A. Congenital tracheal stenosis.
B. Congenital laryngeal cyst.
C. Chronic relapsing polychondritis.
D. Tracheomalacia of the Ellis-van Creveld syndrome.

87. **Persistent horizontal or oblique radiodense lines seen at the base of either lung, referred to as Fleischner lines, are believed due to which of the following except :**
A. Local pleural enfolding and adhesion.
B. Small thromboemboli with subsequent fibrosis.
C. Atelectasis of a pulmonary subsegment and subsequent fibrosis.
D. Linear fibrotic strands as a result of alveolar inflammation.

88. **Concerning bronchial stones, which of the following is most appropriate:**
A. Concretions develop within the bronchi as a result of chronic inflammation.
B. About half of these are found at the root of the right middle lobe bronchus.
C. Most bronchial stones are found in association witht the basal segments of the lower lobes.
D. The stones develop as lymph node calcifications which later perforate into the bronchial lumen.

89. **Regarding PIE (pulmonary infiltrates and eosinophilia), which of the following is least correct :**
A. Asthma is rarely a symptom of this group of diseases.
B. Polyartheritis nodosa is a member of this group.
C. Caplan's syndrome is grouped with PIE.
D. Infection with aspergillus accompanied by asthma is in the PIE definition.

90. **Characteristic feature of chronic mesenteric ischemia is :**
A. Thumb printing
B. Uncoiling of loops
C. Circumferential ulcer
D. Dilatation of gut between strictures

91. **Cortical rim nephrogram is seen in the following except :**
A. Renal vein thrombosis
B. Acute Tubular necrosis
C. Acute total main renal artery obstruction
D. Medullary cystic kidney

Ans.										
	74. D	75. C	76. C	77. B	78. B	79. A	80. C	81. B	82. B	83. A
	84. D	85. C	86. B	87. D	88. B,D	89. C	90. D	91. D		

92. Accordion Corduroyor Honey comb vertebrae are seen in the following except :
A. Multiple myeloma B. Haemangioma
C. Lymphoma D. Fluorosis

93. Agyria or Lissencephaly is :
A. Autosomal dominant B. Autosomal recessive
C. Sex-linked recessive D. Not inherited

94. Following are features of anencephaly except :
A. Exaggerated lordosis
B. Hypoplastic thalami
C. Rachischisis
D. Imperfect formed skull base

95. Brain lipoma is associated most often with agenesis of :
A. C P angle
B. Cerebellomedullary cystern
C. Corpus callosum
D. Pituitary fossa

96. Biological half life of Technetium-99m pertechnetate is :
A. 6 hours B. 24 hours
C. 30 days D. 2 years

97. Double-bubble sign is typically seen in :
A. Trisomy 18 B. Trisomy 21
C. Turner's syndrome D. Klinefelter's syndrome

98. Ruptured ectopic pregnancy with blood in pelvis is classified as type —— spectrum.
A. 1 B. 2
C. 3 D. 4

99. Fetus greater than atleast —— g at term is macrosomia.
A. 3.0 B. 3.5
C. 4.0 D. 5.0

100. Physical half life Gallium-67 citrate is —— days :
A. 3.3 B. 7.2
C. 10.6 D. 15. 2

101. A lactating woman undergone Gallium scintigraphy should stop breast feeding for :
A. 1 week B. 2 weeks
C. 4 weeks D. Not at all

102. On radionuclide esophagram, normal transit time of substance is :
A. 5 sec B. 15 sec
C. 30 sec D. 60 sec

103. 'Moon sign' is seen in :
A. Amoeboma B. Hydatidosis
C. Ca colon D. Volvulus

104. Barber pole sign is midgut volvulus is seen on :
A. Plain film B. Ba meal
C. CT Scan D. Angiography

105. Which of the following is 'Sign of the camalote' in hydatid cyst is :
A. Rupture of pericyst with air
B. Dissection between peri and exocyst
C. Collapsed cyst membrane floating on the fluid
D. Calcification of cyst

106. All substances may be rendered radioactive by the influence of the emanations of radium and substances thus influenced hold their radioactivity longer when enclosed in some material through which emanations cannot pass is —— law.
A. Descartes B. Draper
C. Curie D. Ewald

107. Tail sign in lung is seen in :
A. Bronchiectasis
B. Bronchiolitis obliterans
C. Bronchoalveolar carcinoma
D. Bronchopulmonary fistula

108. Following tumors may metastasize to stomach except :
A. Ca prostate B. Ca kidney
C. Malignant melanoma D. Ca lung

109. Most common cause of Malakoplakia is :
A. Congenital B. Infective
C. Urinary obstruction D. Hyperparathyroidism

110. Mesoblastic nephroma in a fetus can be detected on ultrasonography by :
A. Oligohydramnios
B. Polyhydramnios
C. Hyperechogenic tumor resembling ovarian cyst.
D. Calcified renal mass without distortion of collecting system.

111. Hutchinson's syndrome is characterized by the following except :
A. Primary adr. neuroblastoma
B. Proptosis
C. Extensive skeletal metastasis
D. Massive hepatomegaly

112. Calcification of ear cartilages may be seen in :
A. Hypoparathyroidism B. Hyperthyroidism
C. Addison's disease D. Conn's syndrome

113. In a child, tumor of following may metastasize to testes except :
A. Nephroblastoma B. Neuroblastoma
C. Melanoma D. Ca rectum

114. Double-bubble sign may be seen in following except :
A. Duodenal web
B. Malrotation
C. Preduodenal portal vein
D. Duodenal diverticulum

Ans.									
92. D	93. B	94. B	95. C	96. A	97. B	98. C	99. C	100. A	101. B
102. B	103. B	104. D	105. C	106. C	107. C	108. B	109. B	110. B	111. D
112. C	113. B	114. D							

115. **Gestational sac fills the chorionic cavity by —— weeks.**
A. 7-8 B. 8-9
C. 11-12 D. 14-16

116. **"Threads and Streaks" sign is seen in :**
A. Crohn's disease B. Portal vein thrombosis
C. Congenital megacolon D. Intussusception

117. **Star gazing foetus is seen in :**
A. Erythroblastosis foetalis
B. Down's syndrome
C. Foetal death
D. Rickets

118. **Which is the least common finding among following in rheumatoid lung :**
A. Punctate/nodular densities
B. Reticulonodular densities
C. Pleural thickening
D. Honeycomb lung

119. **Following tumors may spread to breast except :**
A. Malanoma B. Leukaemia
C. Ovarian carcinoma D. Renal cell carcinoma

120. **"Needle shaped" calcification in breast are common in :**
A. Secondaries B. Medullary carcinoma
C. Plasma cell mastitis D. Haematoma of breast

121. **In Down's syndrome, following may be present :**
A. Extra ribs
B. Hypersegmented manubrium
C. Arachnodactyly
D. Pectus excavatum

122. **Right aortic arch is most common in the following congenital heart disease :**
A. Tetralogy of Fallot
B. Tricuspid atresia
C. Transposition of great vessels
D. Truncus arteriosus

123. **Double aortic arch is most often located in :**
A. Right descending aorta
B. Left descending aorta
C. Ascending aorta
D. Aortic arch

124. **Least common cause of chylous ascites in adults is :**
A. Tumor B. Trauma
C. Idiopathic D. Inflammatory

125. **Transient pseudo obstruction is seen in following except :**
A. Scleroderma B. Renal failure
C. CHF D. Electrolyte imbalance

126. **Which of the following is known as 6th ventricle :**
A. Cavum vell interposite
B. Cavum vergae
C. Cavum septi pellucidi
D. Colloid cyst

127. **Which of the following has the highest incidence of "ring blush" on CT :**
A. Glioblastoma B. Grade-II astrocytoma
C. Neurocysticercosis D. Abscess

128. **Low attenuation lesion in basal ganglia may be seen in following except :**
A. Hypoglycemia B. Wilson's disease
C. Methanol intoxication D. Dhatura poisoning

129. **'Fetal head' on ultrasonography can be identified at —— weeks :**
A. 8 B. 10
C. 14 D. 16

130. **99Tcm HIDA shows the normal gall bladder and biliary tract at —— min.**
A. 15 B. 30
C. 60 D. 120

131. **X-ray changes seen in Jaccoud's syndrome are :**
A. Ligamentous calcification
B. Hook like erosions in metacarpal heads
C. Calcification in intervertebral discs
D. Periosteal elevation along shafts of long bones

132. **A rare disorder affecting people between 4 to 20 years with pain in hips or knees called Handigodu syndrome has been reported in India from :**
A. Orissa B. Karnataka
C. TN D. A.P

133. **X-rays in the following disorders are normal except :**
A. Lyme disease
B. Haemochromatosis
C. Henoch Schonlein purpura
D. Metorheostosis

134. **In chronic pancreatitis, cholangiopancreatography shows the following except :**
A. String of pearls
B. Nipping
C. Beading
D. Threads and Streaks sign

135. **Most common site of Malakoplakia is :**
A. Renal Pelvis B. Upper ureter
C. Lower ureter D. Bladder

136. **Ainhum disease or dactylolysis is most common on —— toe.**
A. 1 B. 2
C. 4 D. 5

137. **Barton fracture is fracture of :**
A. Talus B. Radius
C. Ulna D. Fibula

138. **Beak sign on nephrogram is seen in :**
A. Renal duplication B. Renal dysgenesis
C. Renal cyst D. Renal infarction

Ans.									
115. C	116. B	117. B	118. D	119. D	120. C	121. B	122. D	123. B	124. B
125. A	126. B	127. D	128. D	129. C	130. B	131. B	132. B	133. B	134. D
135. D	136. D	137. B	138. C						

139. 'Lemon sign' is seen in skull when abnormality is located in :

A. Sagittal suture B. Coronal suture
C. Cisterna magna D. IV ventricle

140. Nubbin sign is seen in testicular :

A. Trauma B. Torsion
C. Tumor D. Hydrocele

141. In hypotonic duodenography, following is used :

A. Biligraffin B. Insulin
C. Glucagon D. Frusemide

142. In Don's syndrome, which of the following is abnormal :

A. Proximal phalanx of fourth finger
B. Middle phalanx of fourth finger
C. Middle phalanx of fifth finger
D. Proximal phalanx of fifth finger

143. The fields used in MRI in clinical practice is —— tesla.

A. 0.15-1.5 B. 1.5-2.5
C. 2.5-3.5 D. 3.5-4.5

144. Basal ganglia calcification is seen in the following except :

A. Fahr's disease B. Cockayne syndrome
C. Down's syndrome D. Cushing's syndrome

145. Calcification is least common in :

A. Chordoma
B. Pinealoma
C. Pituitary adenoma
D. Choroid plexus papilloma

146. 'Fetal Node' on ultrasound of abdomen can be identified from—— week.

A. 4-5 B. 5-6
C. 6-7 D. 9-10

147. Which of the following frequencies show the best anatomical details in MRI :

A. Spin echo B. Inversion recovery
C. Saturation recovery D. Any of the above

148. Gray scale used to get a more realistic picture of the tissue is a further refinement of ---scan of ultrasonography.

A. A B. B
C. M D. All of the above

149. The substance most widely used in medical ultrasonics is —— zirconate titanate :

A. Silver B. Sodium
C. Magnesium D. Lead

150. Joint most commonly involved by Lymes disease is:

A. Hip B. Knee
C. Ankle D. Shoulder

Ans. **139. B** **140. B** **141. C** **142. C** **143. A** **144. D** **145. C** **146. C** **147. B** **148. B** **149. D** **150. B**

REVIEW PAPER-II

(Based on Difficult & Important MCQ's)

1. **Nelaton's line is also known as —— line :**
A. Sydney B. Roser
C. Ullmann D. Poirier

2. **A method of locating the fissure of Rolando is —— metnod :**
A. Ritgen B. Schafer
C. Schuller D. Thane

3. **The total length of an embryo or fetus in inches for the first five months, equals the numerical sum of the number of the previous lunar months since conception, for the last five lunar months (It equals the product of the number of the month multiplies by 2) is —— rule :**
A. Allen B. Arey
C. Bergmann D. Budin

4. **Paradoxical diaphragm contraction is —— phenomenon :**
A. Hochsinger's B. Kienbock
C. Goldblatt D. Gengou

5. **A zone of metaphyseal degeneration sometimes seen in the bones in infantile scurvy is —— line :**
A. Voigt B. Wagner
C. Trummerfeld D. Sydney

6. **An aneurysm of sinus of valsalva usually arises from :**
A. Posterior aortic sinus B. Right ventricle
C. Left aortic sinus D. Right aortic sinus

7. **Variation in transcardiac measuration on a routine erect teleroentgenogram of the chest between diastole and systole is about —— % :**
A. 1% B. 3%
C. 7% D. 12%

8. **Pirie's bone is an occasionally occurring ossicle found near :**
A. Patella B. Talus
C. Medial malleolus D. Femoral head

9. **The sensitivity of cells to radiation varies directly with the reproductive capacity of the cells and inversely with their degree of differentiation is —— law :**
A. Bunson-Roscoe B. Bergonie - Tribondeau
C. Bastian-Bruns D. Einstein-Starck

10. **The photochemical effect produced is equal to the product of the intensity of the illumination and the duration of exposure is —— law :**
A. Farr B. Ewald's
C. Bunsen-Roscoe D. Behring's

11. **In radiotherapy, the point of origin of a mucous membrane tumor is the last site of heal following irradiation is —— law :**
A. Curie's B. Dollo's
C. Coutard's D. Godelier's

12. **Following are roentgen signs associated with peripheral pulmonary carcinoma except :**
A. Fleischner lines B. Rigler's notch
C. Notch sign D. None of the above

13. **Emphysematous pyelonephritis is most often associated with :**
A. Trauma B. DM
C. SLE D. Renal tubular acidosis

14. **Only the rays that are absorbed by a photochemical substance will produce a chemical change it is —— law :**
A. Donder's B. Draper's
C. Flint's D. Flourens

15. **On usual CT scale of densities (-1000 + 1000), brain tissue would be expected to measure :**
A. -10 to +10 B. 0 to +20
C. +10 to +30 D. +20 to + 45

16. **Lines of retarded growth seen radiographically at the epiphyses of long bones are —— lines :**
A. Corrigan B. Correra
C. Harris D. Hensen's

Ans.	1. C	2. D	3. B	4. B	5. C	6. D	7. C	8. B	9. B	10. C
	11. C	12. D	13. B	14. B	15. D	16. C				

17. For spondylolisthesis, best view is :
A. Anterior oblique B. Posterior oblique
C. A.P. D. Lateral

18. On CT scale of densities, CSF will have density of :
A. 0 B. +15
C. +30 D. +40

19. A line from glabella to pogonion is —— line :
A. Trummerfeld B. Sergent's
C. Retzius's D. Topinard's

20. For orbital emphysema, best view is :
A. Occipitomental B. Occipitofrontal
C. Lateral view D. Any of the above

21. Which of the following conditions can be readily diagnosed by diagnostic ultrasonic techniques :
A. Ca cervix
B. Endometrial carcinoma
C. Uterine leiomyosarcomas
D. Benign fibromyomata

22. Normal biparietal increment is about —— mm/week in 16th-30th week :
A. 1 B. 2
C. 3 D. 4

23. A line in the radiograph of the chest, around the outline of the thorax and bounding the lung fields is —— line :
A. Beudelocque's B. Borsieri's
C. Brucke's D. Correra's

24. Ultrasonic diagnosis of multiple gestation is most accurate at and beyond —— gestation week :
A. 12 B. 13
C. 14 D. 15

25. On ultrasound of endocrine exophthalmos, the earliest sign is enlargement of :
A. Lateral rectus B. Superior rectus
C. Inferior rectus D. Medial rectu

26. A linear shadow on the lateral radiography of the knee, representing tangential bone in the intercondylar space is —— line :
A. Duhot's B. Dobie
C. Blumensaat's D. Ebeth

27. The most specific non invasive technique for diagnosis of endocrine exphthalmos is :
A. CT scan
B. Radionuclide scan
C. Orbital echography
D. MRI

28. Accurate assessment of gestatinal age by ultrasonic measurement of fetal biparietal diameter is best made from —— week :
A. 12-20 B. 15-25
C. 16-30 D. 18-36

29. CT scans of orbit often fail to demonstrate —— rectus muscle :
A. Superior B. Inferior
C. Lateral D. Medial

30. Absence or proximal interruption of right pulmonary artery is often associated with following except :
A. TOF B. PAH
C. PDA D. TS

31. Complete interruption of aortic arch may be associated with :
A. PDA
B. ASD
C. Large descending aorta
D. Hypertension in upper limbs

32. CNS sarcoid often produces which of the following angiographic findings :
A. Small or large vessel occlusion
B. Extravasation
C. Neovascularity
D. Mass effect

33. Metastatic tumors which may present as subarachnoid haemorrhage are following except :
A. Hypernephroma B. Chorio carcinoma
C. Malignant melanoma D. Reticulum cell sarcoma

34. The absorption of energy from radiation in biological material results in ionization releasing which minimum amount of energy :
A. 4.9 eV B. 3.3 eV
C. 33 eV D. 33 MeV

35. Radiation cataracts in humans may be produced by a minimum single gamma ray exposure of —— rads :
A. 50 B. 100
C. 200 D. 1000

36. In pulse echo-mode, the usual clinical ultrasonic transducer receives echoes for how much of the total scan time :
A. 75% B. 95%
C. 99.9% D. 100%

37. A line from glabella to the pogonion is —— line :
A. Wagner B. Ulmann
C. Topinard D. Thompson

Ans.									
17. B	18. B	19. D	20. A	21. D	22. C	23. D	24. D	25. C	26. C
27. C	28. C	29. B	30. D	31. A	32. D	33. D	34. C	35. C	36. C
37. C									

38. **Of the biological materials usually examined by ultrasound, sound passes slowest through :**
A. Bone B. Blood
C. Gas D. Muscle

39. **The axial line of the big toe which if extended passes through the centre of the heel of shoes have never been worn is —— line :**
A. Hunter B. Meyer
C. Feiss D. Duhot

40. **'Fogging phenomenon' is seen in :**
A. Appendicular abscess B. Ac. Pancreatitis
C. Cerebral infarction D. Ac. Cholecystitis

41. **Lines of retarded growth seen radiographically at the epiphyses of long bones are ——— lines :**
A. Feiss B. Harris
C. Kaes D. Moyer

42. **Which of the following is wrongly matched for MRI appearance of haemorrhage :**

	T1	T2
A. Oxyhemoglobin	High	High
B. Hemosiderin	Low	Low
C. Oedema	Iso	High
D. Fibrous tissue	High	Low

43. **A prominent line on the promontary of the sacrum is known as ———line :**
A. Correra B. Brucke
C. Kilian D. Morgan

44. **Following are true about CNS changes in Krabbe disease except :**
A. High density lesions
B. Brain atrophy
C. White matter involved
D. Ventricular enlargement

45. **Rarest intracranial glioma is :**
A. Astroblastoma
B. Spongioblastoma polare
C. Oligodendroglioma
D. Globlastoma

46. **Which of the following is true about vertebral artery :**
A. Right is usually greater than left
B. Left may arise directly from aorta
C. Originates from Aortic arch
D. Enters transverse foramina at C5

47. **A line in the radiograph of the chest around the outline of the thorax and bounding the lung fields is —— line :**
A. Borsieri B. Duhot
C. Correra D. Gottinger

48. **A pathological condition in the newborn skull which will probably require immediate attention is :**
A. Cranium bifidum frontalis
B. Parietal foramina
C. Convolutional markings
D. Bathrocephaly

49. **Congenital fetal abnormalities may be most expected when exposure to radiation occurs during ——— week following conception :**
A. First B. 1-2
C. 2-4 D. 4-8

50. **Least common site of berry aneurysm among following is :**
A. Middle cerebral
B. Carotid bifurcation
C. Ant. Communicating artery
D. Post. Communicating artery

51. **Lactoferrin has been demonstrated in the following tumors except one known to localize gallium-67 :**
A. Hodgkin's lymphoma
B. Melanoma
C. ALL
D. Burkitt's lymphoma

52. **Which is the least common cause of photon deficient lesion seen on bone scan :**
A. Sickle cell anemia
B. Osteomyelitis
C. Multiple myeloma
D. Bronchogenic carcinoma secondaries

53. **The severity of reaction to intravenous administration of iodinated contrast media is not related to which of the following :**
A. Speed of injection
B. Type of iodinated contrast
C. Antihistamine used as premedication
D. All of the above

54. **Which of the following is least likely to be confused with pancreatic pseudocyst on CT-scan or ultrasonography :**
A. Pancreatic cystadenoma
B. Pancreatic cystadenocarcinoma
C. Pancreatic phlegmon
D. None of the above

55. **Decay per second is called :**
A. 1 Sievert B. 10 Sievert
C. 1 Becquerel D. 10 Becquerels

Ans.									
38. C	39. B	40. C	41. B	42. D	43. C	4. A	45. A	46. B	47. C
48. C	49. C	50. B	51. C	52. C	53. D	54. C	55. C		

56. Space between the pericardium and the beginning of the aorta is —— space :
A. Zang's B. Westberg's
C. Nuel's D. Larrey's

57. The middle space of the three clear lung fields in the radiograph of the chest in oblique projection when the rays pass from left posteriorly to the right anteriorly is —— space :
A. Henke's B. Douglas
C. Holtzknecht's D. Czermak's

58. A ring shaped shadow observed in a radiograph of the skull, caused by an aneurysm of a cerebral artery is —— ring :
A. Albl's B. Balbianis
C. Bickel's D. Duran's

59. In the radiograph after a barium meal, a narrow area or focal contraction of the mid third of the transverse colon representing the junction of primitive midgut and hindgut and marking an area of overlap between the superior and inferior nerve plexues is —— ring :
A. Cannon's B. Carpentier
C. Duran D. Liesegang

60. The view used for demonstrating fractures and malformations of the temporomandibular joint is —— view :
A. Kraske B. Mayer
C. Rose's D. Valentine

61. A semi recumbent position of the patient for radiography as a means of determining the diametes of the superior strait of the pelvis —— position :
A. Albert B. Casselberry
C. Duncan D. Elliot

62. A line from nasion to lamba is —— line :
A. Zollner B. Wagner's
C. Virchow D. Sydney

63. The metastasis of mesothelioma is most common to :
A. Ipsilateral lung B. Contralateral lung
C. Mediastinal nodes D. Pleura

64. If there is interstial edema and no alveolar edema, Mitral stenosis is staged as :
A. 1 B. 2
C. 3 D. 4

65. A significant radiographic characteristic associated with the niche of the typical benign gastric ulcer in profile is —- line :
A. Harris B. Hensen's
C. Morgan's D. Hampton

66. For assessing CPD best view is —— :
A. Oblique B. A.P.
C. PA D. Lateral

67. Newton's ringing (concentric) artefacts in the CT image of a third or fourth generation device are most likely due to :
A. Patient motion
B. Asynchronous motion of gantry during scanning
C. Surgical metallic clips
D. Imbalanced detectors

68. A curved line seen in radiographs of skull, indicating the position of the optic groove is —— line:
A. Gottinger B. Granger's
C. Hensen's D. Holden's

69. Following has a negative CT number :
A. Bone B. Gas
C. Metal D. Water

70. Muller maneuver is used to :
A. Increase size of pulmonary vessels
B. Decrease size of pulmonary vessels
C. Increase size of heart
D. Decrease size of spleen

71. The minimum size of polyp that can be consistently identified in roentgen examination is —— in diameter :
A. 0.3-0.7 B. 0.7-1.0
C. 1.2-1.5 D. 1.7-2.0

72. On the usual CT scale of densities (-1000 to + 1000), CSF would be expected to measure :
A. -10 B. +15
C. +25 D. +35

73. A dose of rads said to produce sterility in females is —— of that in males :
A. One third B. Half
C. Equal D. Double

74. Only those rays of ultraviolet light that are absorbed produce a chemical effect is —— law :
A. Laplace B. Gudden's
C. Grotthus D. Haeckel

75. Flexion, abduction and outward rotation of thigh in coxitis is —— position :
A. Albert's B. Bonner's
C. Bozeman's D. English

76. A radiographic position which gives an oblique view of the zygomatic arch projected free of superimposed structures is —— position :
A. Jones B. Fuch's
C. Simons D. Mayer

Ans.	56. B	57. C	58. A	59. A	60. B	61. A	62. C	63. A	64. B	65. D
	66. D	67. D	68. B	69. B	70. A	71. B	72. B	73. B	74. C	75. B
	76. B									

77. A straight line connecting the medial epicondyle of the humerus with the top of the olecranon when the arm is extended is ——— line :
A. Eberth's B. Duhot
C. Hueter D. Meyer

78. A curved line seen in radiographs of skulls, indicating the position of the optic groove is ——— line :
A. Harris B. Granger
C. Gottinger D. Holden

79. 'Thumbprinting' may be seen in :
A. Midgut volvulus
B. Acute amobiasis
C. Pneumatosis intestinalis
D. Crohn's disease
E. None of the above

80. Horseshoe or boonerang configuration of brain is seen in —— holoprosencephaly :
A. Alobar B. Semilobar
C. Lobar D. All of the above

81. "Ash leaf patches or spermint patches" are seen in :
A. SLE B. Scleroderma
C. Tuberous sclerosis D. Venous angioma

82. Ask-Upmark kidney is seen in :
A. Congenital renal hypoplasia
B. Conn syndrome
C. Chronic GN
D. Wilm's tumor

83. Askin tumor arises from :
A. VI nerve B. Intercostal nerve
C. Costochondral cartilage D. Diaphragm

84. Groundglass appearance of vertebra is seen in :
A. Paget disease
B. Eosinophilic granuloma
C. Aneurysmal bone cyst
D. Fibrous dysplasia

85. 'Asomia' is abnormality in :
A. I nerve B. Olfactory lobe
C. Pleura D. Vertebra

86. Asterisk sign on CT scan is seen in :
A. Legg-Perthes-Calve disease
B. Leukemia of bone
C. Reticulum cell sarcoma
D. Malignant fibrous histiocytoma

87. Juvenile pilocytic astrocytoma arises from :
A. Pons B. Medulla
C. Thalamus D. Optic nerve

88. A1 and A2 segments are of —— artery :
A. Ant. cerebral B. Middle cerebral
C. Post. cerebral D. Vertebral

89. Mother-in-law phenomenon is seen in :
A. IVP
B. OCG
C. Cerebral angiography
D. Hystero-salpingography

90. Atypical meningioma is ———shaped :
A. Sigma B. Curvilinear
C. Comma D. Delta

91. Soap bubble appearance is seen in :
A. Mesenteric ischemia
B. Meconium ileus
C. Ca colon
D. Diverticulosis of colon

92. Gas in bowel wall is seen in the following except :
A. Gastric pneumatosis B. Phlegmonous gastritis
C. Endoscopy D. Diverticulitis

93. Picket fencing in Barium is seen in :
A. Muconium plug syndrome
B. TB Mesenteritis
C. Mesenteric ischemia
D. Mesenteric cyst

94. Regarding tracheal neoplasms, which of the following is the least accurate statement ?
A. Most tracheal neoplasms are submucosal
B. Of the tracheal neoplasms, the papillomas are likely to become malignant
C. Tracheal scleromas and some amyloid tumors may be radiographically similar to benign tracheal neoplasms
D. Most tracheal neoplasms in adults are benign

95. Which of the following conditions is not associated with recurrent pneumothoraces ?
A. Endometriosis B. Apical pulmonary bulla
C. Histiocytosis X D. None of the above

96. Calcification in pulmonary metastases may be found most commonly in which of the following ?
A. Chondrosarcoma
B. Thyroid carcinoma
C. Osteogenic sarcoma
D. Ovarian cystadenocarcinoma

97. A decrease in functional residual capacity (FRC) is associated with all of the following except :
A. Diffuse pulmonary fibrosis
B. Alveolar microlithiasis
C. Ascites
D. Bronchial asthma

Ans.									
77 C	78. B	79. ALL	80. A	81. C	82. A	83. B	84. D	85. D	86. A
87. D	88. A	89. C	90. C	91. B	92. D	93. C	94. D	95. D	96. C
97. D									

98. Shaver's disease is characterized by all of the following except :

A. It develops after only months (not years) of chronic exposure
B. It is a form of silicosis
C. It is complicated by bullous emphysema and spontaneous pneumothorax
D. It is due to daily exposure to tiny, cut hairs from dryshaving (as with an electric razor)

99. In the roentgen appearance of the lungs following near drowning, which of the following is least likely ?

A. The pattern is that of pumonary edema
B. The findings tend to be bilaterally symmetrical
C. Resolution of the rentogen findings is usually within a week
D. If the near-drowning was in sea water, there is considerably less edema than if in fresh water

100. Which of the following roentgen signs is not associated with peripheral pulmonary carcinoma ?

A. Fleischner line
B. Increase in size over an interval of time
C. Lubulated nodule (notch sign)
D. None of the above

101. The diagnosis of bronchiolar carcinoma is unlikely if which of the following conditions prevail except :

A. If the pulmonary lesion becomes increasingly demarcated with time
B. If the lesion shows persistent decrease in size or density
C. If the lesion is associated with lymph node enlargement
D. None of the above

102. Complete interruption of the aortic arch may be associted with :

A. Ventricular septal defect
B. Hypertension in upper arms
C. Large ascending aorta
D. None of the above

103. Marfan's syndrome is characterized by the following findings except :

A. Dilatation of the sinuses of Valsalva
B. Arachnodactlyly
C. Frequent association with dissecting aneurysms of the ascending aorta
D. Obstruction by narrowing of the renal arteries, especially on the left

104. Tricuspid atresia is associated with following except:

A. Pulmonary stenosis
B. A right-to left-atrial shunt
C. Severely underdeveloped right ventricle
D. Normal-sized heart

105. Unusually small cardiac size, as noted in routine PA chest X-ray examination, may be due to :

A. Dehydration B. Bronchial asthma
C. Addison's disease D. All of the above

106. Pompe's disease is characterized by :

A. Possible sudden death in the first year of life from conduction abnormalities
B. An acute myocarditis
C. No cardiomegaly
D. A relationship to systemic glycogen storage disease

107. Variation in transcardiac mensuration on a routine erect teleroentgenogram of the chest between diastole and systole is about :

A. 1-3% B. 5-10%
C. 10-15% D. 15-20%

108. An aneurysm of the sinus of Valsalva usually arises from the :

A. Left aortic sinus
B. Right aortic sinus
C. Posterior aortic sinus
D. Pulmonary outflow tract

109. Squatting is a common clinical observation in patients with congenital heart disease. A suggested reason for this posture is :

A. The peripheral resistance is raised increasing systemic venous return. This, in turn, reduces the volume of left-right shunting with increase in arterial oxygenation
B. Lowering the center of body mass reduces the cardiac effort to maintain flow to the brain
C. Compression of abdominal contents and flexing of the thighs reduce flow to the lower part of the body reducing cardiac effort
D. Many of these patients fatigue easily and squatting represents a natural method of resting without reclining

110. Regarding mycotic aneurysms of the aorta, which of the following is correct?

A. These aneurysms enlarge slowly
B. A source of infection is usually not idendifiable
C. Due to the infective nature, these are not amenable to surgical repair
D. Right-sided bacterial endocarditis as a source of mycotic aneurysms is particularly prevalent in drug addicts

Ans. 98. D 99. D 100. D 101. D 102. A 103. D 104. D 105. D 106. A 107. B 108. B 109. A 110. D

111. Pseudocoarctation of the aorta is best described by which of the following ?

A. A mild narrowing of the aortic lumen at the level of the ligamentum arteriosum

B. A narrowing of the aortic ring with valvular insufficiency and poststenotic dilatation of the ascending aorta

C. A narrowing of the aorta at the level of the brachiocephalic vessel to the right, often related to a large atheromatous plaque

D. A kinking or buckling of the aortic arch which simulates the plain film findings of true aortic coarctation

112. The term, pulmonary sling, refers to :

A. Distal origin of the right pulmonary artery

B. Dysphagia from pressure of the aberrant artery

C. Persistent ligamentum arteriosum which compresses the left main-stem bronchus in a sling-like manner

D. Origin of the left pulmonary artery from either the right pulmonary artery or the distal main pulmonary artery

113. The Law, Stenvers, and Owen radiographic projections are used to demonstrate :

A. Facial structures

B. Lateal ventricules in pneumoencephalography

C. The temporal bone

D. The atlanto-occipital articulation

114. Which of the following is not associated with nasal septal destruction ?

A. Sarcoidosis

B. Benign nasal polyps

C. Midline lethal granuloma

D. Osteomata

115. Radiation cataract in humans may be produced by a minimum single gamma ray exposure of ------ rods :

A. 25-50 B. 50-100

C. 100-200 D. 200-500

116. Which of the following is not a good estimate of basilar impression ?

A. Chamberlain's line B. Bull's angle

C. Bimastoid line D. Basal angle

117. Which of the following is do not ordinarily cause membranous intracranial calcification except :

A. Arteriovenous malformation

B. Acute subdural hematoma

C. Agyria

D. Tuberculous meningitis

118. The most common acute CT finding in the head of an abused child is :

A. Old or new skull fracture

B. Acute interhemispheric subdural hematoma

C. Posterior fossa subdural hematoma

D. Epidural hematoma

119. A pathological condition in the newborn skull which will probably require immediate attention is :

A. Bathrocephaly

B. Caput succedaneum

C. Cranium bifidum frontalis

D. Convolutional markings

120. CNS sarcoid may produce which of the following angiographic findings?

A. Small vessel occlusions

B. Extravasation

C. Neovascularity

D. Mass effect

121. Which of the following are not CT signs of the Chiari II malformation?

A. The third ventricle is large

B. The fourth ventricle is not visualized or appears small

C. Scalloping of the posterior surface of the petrous pyramids

D. Falx hypoplasia

122. The Dandy-Walker syndrome includes all of the following except :

A. Ths malformation is due to agenesis of the formina of Magendie and Luschka

B. Dysgenesis of the vermia

C. Posterior fossa cyst communication with a dilated fourth ventricle

D. Elevation of the torcular Herophili

123. Severe chest pain with hematemesis and dysphagia, in association with mediastinal emphysema, is characteristic of :

A. Ruptured esophageal varices

B. Mallory-Weiss syndrome

C. Boerhaave syndrome

D. Intramural esophageal rupture

124. Regarding suspected toxic megacolon, which of the following is least likely ?

A. Barium enema may be useful in order to demonstrate the shaggy mucosal ulcerations

B. The most commonly associated disease is ulcerative colitis

C. The greatest gaseous distention is in the transverse colon

D. The incidence of bowel wall perforation of high

Ans. 111. D 112. D 113. C 114. D 115. D 116. D 117. D 118. B 119. D 120. D
121. A 122. A 123. C 124. A

125. Concerning the prune belly (Eagle Barret) syndrome, which of the following is least likely ?
A. This condition is related to fetal abdominal distention leading to decreased or absent abdominal musculature
B. Males and females are afflicted in nearly equal proportion
C. Many of these infants have multiple, associated anomalies in other organ systems
D. There is most often either uretheral obstruction or failure to empty the bladder

126. Identification of normal thymus on frontal x-ray of the chest can be made more positive by following except :
A. Steroid therapy B. Sail sign
C. Wavy thymus sign D. None of the above

127. What is the best way to describe the relationship of the following nuclides ?
$^{23}_{11}Na$ $^{24}_{12}Mg$
A. Isotopic B. Isomeric
C. Isoenergic D. Isotonic

128. The focal spot size of an x-ray tube is best measured by :
A. Exposure with step-wedge device
B. Pin-hole camera
C. Spinning top
D. Wire mesh exposure

129. Radiation leakage from the housing of a diagnostic x-ray tube operated at the limit of mA and kVp should be no more than :
A. 10 mR/hr at 1 m B. 50 mR/hr at 1 m
C. 100 mR/hr at 1 m D. 200 mR/hr at 1 m

130. Shenton's line is also known as ——— line :
A. Roland B. Skinner
C. Poirier D. Spieghel

131. Scattered radiation from a fluoroscopic procedure is increased by —— % when the area being exposed to the X-ray beam is increased from a field of 3cm x 3 cm to 5 cm x 5 cm :
A. 100 B. 150
C. 200 D. 300

132. In cae of blawout fractures, which of the following is most likely fractured :
A. Inferior rim of ipsilateral orbit
B. Ant. wall of ipsilateral maxillary sinus
C. Zygomatic arch
D. Greater wing of sphenoid

133. Which of the following is not a good estimate of the basilar impression :
A. Chamberlain's line B. Basal angle
C. Bull's angle D. Bimastoid line

134. The most common acute CT finding in the head of an abused child is :
A. Skull fracture
B. Epidural haematoma
C. Acute interhemispheric subdural haema-toma
D. Posterior fossa subdural haematoma

135. Moon sign is seen in :
A. Hydatid disease B. Cysticercosis
C. Duodenal atresia D. Volvulus

136. Fracture of bronchus is most common at :
A. At carina
B. Distal to carina right side
C. Proximal to carina left side
D. Proximal to carina right side

137. Extramedullary plasmacytoma is common in :
A. Trachea B. Upper nose
C. Conjunctiva D. Lymph nodes

138. The correct sequence of carcinogenic potential of following (in decreasing order) is :
I. Amosite II. Chrysotile
III. Antophyllite IV. Crocidolite
A. I, II, III, IV B. I, III,IV, II
C. IV, III, II, I D. IV, I, II, III

139. Sign of Camalote is seen in :
A. Hepatoma B. Hirschsprung's disease
C. Hydatidosis D. Turner's syndrome

140. Osteitis condensans ilii is found mainly in following :
A. Trauma B. Pregnancy
C. Fluorosis D. Ankylosing spondylitis

141. New bone formation is common in the following except :
A. Osteoarthritis B. Rheumatoid arthritis
C. Reiter's syndrome D. Psoriatic arthritis

142. Most typical bone changes in sarcoidosis are seen in :
A. Phalanges B. Ribs
C. Skull D. Spine

143. In the Salter-Harris classification of epiphyseal injuries, which of the following is least likely to be identified on immediate radiographic examination :
A. II B. III
C. IV D. V

Ans.	125. B	126. D	127. D	128. B	129. C	130. C	131. D	132. B	133. B	134. C
	135. A	136. B	137. A	138. D	139. C	140. B	141. B	142. A	143. D	

144. Variation in transcardiac mensuration on a routine erect teleroentgenogram of the chest between diastole and systole is about :

A. 0-4 B. 5-10

C. 15-20 D. Above 20

145. Calcification in pulmonary metastases may be found most commonly in :

A. Thyroid carcinoma B. Ca breast

C. Chondrosarcoma D. Osteosarcoma

146. Figure '3' sign is present in :

A. Turner's syndrome B. Trilogy of fallot

C. Uhl's anomaly D. Scimitar syndrome

147. The Law, Stenvers and Owen radiographic projections are used to demonstrate :

A. Facial structures

B. Temporal bone

C. The occiput

D. Atlanto occipital articulation

148. An aneurysm of the sinus of Valsalva usually arises from :

A. Left aortic sinus B. Right aortic sinus

C. Posterior aortic sinus D. Right ventricle

149. Radiation leakage from the housing of a diagnostic X-ray tube operated at the limit of mA and kVp should be no more than —— mR/hour at 1m :

A. 50 B. 100

C. 200 D. 300

150. Estimation of fetal maturity by biparietal sonic measurement is accurate to within —— days :

A. +7-10 B. +10-14

C. +12-18 D. +14-21

Ans. 144. B 145. D 146. A 147. B 148. B 149. B 150. A

RADIOLOGY

References Quoted

S.No.	Books
1.	Sutton's **Textbook of Radiology & Imaging.** Churchill Livingstone, New York
2.	Bailey & Love's **Short Practice of Surgery** ELBS, London
3.	Harrison's **Principles of Internal Medicine** McGraw-Hill, New York
4.	Bhatia's **Quick Medical Text Review Series (Radiology)** CBS Publishers & Distributors Pvt. Ltd., Delhi.

Unforgetable Supplement

Bhatia's **Quick Medical Text Review Series** (Quick revision of all the subjects in short time. No need to underline the books read important points). CBS Publishers & Distributors Pvt. Ltd., Delhi.